TALKING ABOUT MIS

SARAH MURPHY grew up in I
now lives in Sussex. She is n
children. Her career experiences i ....ꜱ,
playgroup supervision and teaching, but she now
works as part-time secretary to her husband Pat and
divides her remaining time between her family and
her two main hobbies of writing and riding. She is also
the author of *Coping with Cot Death* (Sheldon 1990).

Overcoming Common Problems Series

For a full list of titles please contact
Sheldon Press, Marylebone Road, London NW1 4DU

Overcoming Common Problems

TALKING ABOUT MISCARRIAGE

Sarah Murphy

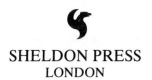

SHELDON PRESS
LONDON

First published in Great Britain in 1992
Sheldon Press, SPCK, Marylebone Road, London NW1 4DU

British Library Cataloguing-in-Publication Data
A catalogue record for this book is available from the British Library
ISBN 0–85969–642–1

Photoset by Deltatype Ltd, Ellesmere Port, Cheshire
Printed in Great Britain by Biddles Ltd, Guildford and King's Lynn

Contents

Acknowledgements   vi

1   Miscarriage – The Facts   1

2   The Physical Impact   17

3   The Emotional Impact   36

4   Coping From Within   45

5   Coping As A Family   61

6   Who Can Help?   72

7   How The Medical Profession Can Help   85

8   Another Baby?   102

Useful Addresses   114

Further reading   119

Index   120

Acknowledgements

I am very grateful to my family and friends for their patience and support, to all those in the health and welfare professions who so kindly assisted and to all those bereaved by miscarriage who so willingly contributed to the book by sharing their experiences. To all those who have been launched on to the road of grieving and self-discovery by the experience of miscarriage and to all those associated personally or professionally who want to know how best to respond and give assistance on the journey, I dedicate this book and hope that it will help.

Sarah Murphy
December 1991

1

Miscarriage – The Facts

When we make plans, they are usually optimistic, positive ones. For those of us who want to have children and create a family, the future that we imagine for ourselves contains a baby and fulfilment and happiness – not unplanned and unexpected pain and loss and grieving. When we experience miscarriage it is a profound shock and one that places us at odds with our own bodies. Often this leads us to a loss of confidence both in our bodies and in ourselves, as well as in a life that suddenly holds for us a harsh awareness that there are no certainties and no guarantees.

Whereas medically miscarriage may seem a trivial event, for those of us who experience it the effects can be both wide-reaching and long-lasting: it not only destroys the reality of our awaited baby, it also destroys all the hopes and plans that accompanied that reality.

This book is intended for those who have found themselves having to cope with miscarriage, whether single or repeated. It is based on my own experiences (one very late miscarriage at 27 weeks and one very early one at about 8 weeks) as well as on the experiences of many others. I hope that it will offer guidance on how to cope with both the immediate effects and the long-term implications and that it will offer insights to families, friends and professionals wanting to know how best to respond and help.

Compared to previous centuries, we live in an age of enhanced standards of living and of medical care, but these very improvements can lull us into assuming that each pregnancy will result in a healthy, full-term baby to receive all the love we are waiting and wanting to give. Consequently, when pregnancy goes wrong and there is no baby, we can feel cheated at a very deep level indeed. Many of us do not even realize how much of ourselves we are investing in our pregnancy until it ends so harshly and abruptly. Afterwards we are unlikely to be able to view either ourselves or the world around us in quite the same way again. We learn much about ourselves, certainly, but the cost is high. I would like this book to serve as a tribute to the courage, strength and resilience of so many women who find themselves having to cope with miscarriage. In their ability to mourn and yet move on and grow from the experience and in their readiness to undertake future pregnancies – despite the risks and anxieties involved – so many women act as a hope and inspiration to all those wanting and needing a baby of their own to love.

This book is intended to answer questions, provide information and offer guidelines on how to cope with the effects of miscarriage. With these points in mind, I have divided the book into eight chapters, but they do not have to be read in the order in which they are presented. This chapter and the next one are factual, but if facts are not what you want to read just now and you are having to cope with the severe emotional impact which often follows a miscarriage, you may prefer to begin with Chapters 3 and 4. Because it is useful to be able to recognize and understand what is known about the causes and possible means of prevention of miscarriage, however, examining the facts does seem the appropriate way to begin.

What soon became apparent when I started investigating the occurrence of miscarriage is the comparative lack of research and information on the subject. This appears to be because, from the medical viewpoint, miscarriage is a very common, routine and usually self-righting event. When finances and resources are so limited, it is understandable that the Health Service is reluctant to channel funds in a direction where the problem usually sorts itself out in the fullness of time. But unfortunately, such a viewpoint takes no account of the physical and emotional trauma suffered by many women who undergo a single or repeated miscarriage, and therefore one of the aims of this book will be to show how and where women's needs are not being met and to make suggestions for improvements in the future.

There is no disputing the fact that miscarriage is very common, although statistics vary depending on when a pregnancy is taken to have started. A considerable number of very early miscarriages go completely unrecognized because the women concerned assume that what they are experiencing is simply a late, heavy period. Obviously if pregnancy is dated from the time of fertilization of the egg by the sperm, or even from the time of implantation, then the rate of miscarriage is going to be higher than if it is dated from the time of the first missed period and the onset of pregnancy symptoms such as breast tenderness or morning sickness. Consequently, figures for miscarriage vary from 1 in 6 pregnancies to as high as 4 in 6, but the most generally accepted view seems to be that about 1 in 5 pregnancies will end in miscarriage. This statistic means that every year thousands of women find themselves having to cope with the experience of miscarriage and its physical and emotional aftermath. This book is intended for all those who feel a sense of loss, no matter at what stage the pregnancy was perceived to have started nor at what stage it ended, prematurely. One of the discoveries I soon made when talking to women who had suffered miscarriage is that the stage of pregnancy at which the miscarriage took place does not necessarily determine the depth of loss and mourning which is felt afterwards. Many women have said to me that those around them seemed to mete out sympathy in direct proportion to the length of pregnancy involved, giving most after a late miscarriage and least after an early one, despite the fact that an early loss can be just as devastating as a late loss. Much seems to depend on the amount of emotional investment in the pregnancy. If the baby was perceived as real, no matter how early on in gestation, then the loss will be very real, too.

The fact that miscarriage is so common does nothing to reduce the impact which it can have, nor to remove the feeling of being very isolated and the only person ever to be coping with such an experience. (At such times it can be very helpful to talk to others who have also experienced miscarriage, either via one of the local support groups of the Miscarriage Association or the National Childbirth Trust or by talking to friends. Miscarriage still tends to be an unspoken subject, but when you do acknowledge it by talking about what has happened, it is surprising how many people will then respond by talking about their own past experience of miscarriage or that of someone close to them. In other words, you do not need to feel that you are alone, an unwilling exception to the rules of motherhood, because many, many others have been through a similar trauma and may well be able to help you.)

Why did it happen?

One of the greatest needs following a miscarriage is for an explanation of why it happened, and one of the harsh facts that mothers find themselves facing is that many miscarriages simply do not have an explanation. Naturally, having experienced one miscarriage the fear is that any future pregnancy may result in miscarriage as well, and it is natural to feel that knowing the cause of the first might help to indicate whether future pregnancies could also be at risk. When an explanation *can* be given, this may help or it may just lead the women concerned to want to say: 'Yes, but what caused the cause?' When no explanation can be found, women are left in a kind of limbo, no longer trusting their own bodies. Although I will be looking at 27 different explanations which have been cited as possible causes of miscarriage, the reality is that in most cases, no cause can be found or attributed with any degree of certainty. When we miscarry, it is very tempting to seize on all the causes which have ever been suggested and to try to make one or more of them fit our own particular experience, even in the absence of any supporting evidence. Although it can be very helpful to be aware of causes which have been cited in the past, I hope you will be able to use the following details as an information source and not as a potential source of worry or guilt. The absence of any obvious cause often leads women to attribute one of their own (no matter how unlikely it may seem) and to blame themselves accordingly. The fact that such a sense of guilt is unwarranted does not prevent it from arising. As many women do find themselves having to cope with feelings of self-blame afterwards, this important reaction will receive attention throughout (see under 'guilt' in index).

Chromosomal Abnormalities

In the absence of any proof, it can be difficult to accept the platitude: 'Nature knows best'. Nevertheless, statistics show that between 50 and 60 per cent of early miscarriages are known to take place because the mother's body is expelling a fetus with chromosomal abnormalities, and the figure is probably higher because some abnormalities are not yet detectable. The alternative would be a full-term baby born either dead or handicapped because of some defect or damage in either the sperm or the ovum (the mother's egg). Such damage can occur before, during or after conception. Although rationally we may be able to accept that miscarriage is the right course of action for our bodies to take in such circumstances, this does not in any way reduce our sense of loss and of being cheated when the miscarriage occurs.

One of the greatest of all miracles is the genetic blueprinting which goes into the making of a baby, which makes each and every one of us so individual and which therefore causes such distress when our unique, irreplaceable baby-to-be does not survive. We all have 46 chromosomes, arranged in 23 pairs inside the nucleus of every cell, with one of each pair being inherited from each parent. It is one thing to make such a statement, quite another to try and

4

visualize the concept – 46 chromosomes within every cell in our bodies. There are two notable exceptions to this rule: the egg cells of the female and the sperm cells of the male, contain only 23 chromosomes each. When the egg and the sperm join at conception, the two sets of 23 chromosomes pair up so that the fertilized egg then has 46 chromosomes. The chromosomes transmit basic genetic characteristics such as height, colour of hair, colour of eyes, the sex of the baby (two x chromosomes coming together will produce a girl, an x and a y chromosome coming together will produce a boy) and so forth. Naturally this is a very vulnerable time, hence the high rate of early miscarriage when damage occurs to otherwise healthy chromosomes or when defective chromosomes pair up at conception. There are many kinds of chromosomal abnormality, some of which can be detected by conducting tests on small fragments of tissue. With some severe abnormalities, the pregnancies will always miscarry, but with some abnormalities such as Down's syndrome and Turner's syndrome, miscarriage may not take place (the rate is 75 per cent for Down's syndrome and 95 per cent for Turner's syndrome).

Usually chromosome abnormalities are 'one-off' accidents during the formation of the individual egg and sperm cells, but very occasionally a parent may carry what is known as a 'balanced chromosome abnormality', which leads to the repeated formation of chromosomally abnormal eggs or sperm resulting in a higher risk of having miscarriages or a chromosomally abnormal baby (this condition accounts for repeated miscarriage in only about 5 per cent of couples). In such cases it is possible to have a chromosome test and therefore anyone finding herself coping with repeated miscarriages should ask for this test for both herself and her partner.

Chromosomal abnormality is one area where more research would be very welcome. At present it is not known how most of these abnormalities arise, and although some feel that exposure to irradiation, for example, may increase the risk, no clear statistical evidence is available. What *is* known is that the chromosomal abnormality known as 'trisomy' increases with age and that trisomy accounts for half of all chromosome abnormalities.

The main chromosome abnormalities following conception (bearing in mind that each individual egg and sperm should itself contain 23 chromosomes) are:

trisomy: one extra chromosome per cell, making 47

monosomy: one chromosome too few per cell, making 45
triploidy: a complete extra set of chromosomes per cell, making 69 (i.e. 23 + 23 + 23)
tetraploidy: twice the normal number of chromosomes, making 92

Non-chromosomal factors

Even when the chromosomes and genes are normal (each chromosome contains thousands of genes), the anatomical structure of the fetus may fail to develop correctly, as in spina bifida (in which the spinal cord does not develop properly). Studies suggest that half of all fetuses which develop spina bifida miscarry spontaneously and consequently the rate of spina bifida in live births is only about 1.7 per 1,000 births.

Maternal problems

Abnormalities of anatomy

Malformations of the uterus (womb) are thought to be present in anywhere between 1 in 1,000 and 2 in 100 women – a wide variance. Some, of course, do not affect the pregnancy in any way but in others the abnormality may be sufficient to adversely affect the blood supply to the placenta or to cause problems for the growing fetus. Thus, miscarriage in the first three months (trimester) of pregnancy does not seem to be increased but in the second trimester the frequency does increase (as many as 25–50 per cent of pregnancies in women with double uteruses are lost at this time). Any woman miscarrying at this stage should therefore ask for a medical examination to exclude anatomical abnormality as a cause. If such an abnormality is found, it is sometimes possible for surgical correction to be carried out. The same holds true for cervical incompetence (where the neck of the uterus relaxes too early, making it impossible for the uterus to retain the baby). If investigation proves this to be the case, then a purse-string stitch can be inserted into the cervix during the next pregnancy to try and reduce the risk of miscarriage.

Fibroids

Fibroids are benign tumours of the uterus. About 20 per cent of all women have one or more present at some time, and usually they do not cause any problem. When fibroids are discovered following a miscarriage it is difficult to know whether or not they have acted as a contributory cause; equally disheartening is that there is little evidence to show whether their removal reduces the risk of further miscarriage.

Polycystic ovaries

When a woman has polycystic ovaries, this results in abnormal levels of the hormone known as luteinizing hormone and this could be significant concerning the potential risk of miscarriage. Work is being carried out at St Mary's Hospital in London and it is hoped that this may lead to encouraging results for women affected in this way.

Hormonal problems

These can cause problems in early pregnancy and they can cause placental failure, which occurs when there are insufficient hormones to keep the placenta in good working order. Progesterone and HCG (human chorionic gonadotrophin) are important hormones involved in the establishment and maintenance of a pregnancy and therefore, in cases of recurring miscarriages where the woman is believed to have a deficient production of such hormones, some doctors advocate hormonal supplementation as a preventive measure. Evidence is lacking, however, as to both the effectiveness and safety of such treatment. A success rate does seem to be achieved in a number of cases, but then over 60 per cent of women are known to have a healthy baby even after three miscarriages and without receiving treatment of any kind, and some studies suggest that placebos (dummy medicines) can be just as beneficial as the hormone supplements. (A placebo is often used in controlled trials. It is known to have no medical effect and can therefore act as a balance to the medical treatment being tested. If, as in the case of miscarriage, it proves to be as beneficial as the active medical treatment, this suggests that the support and interest accompanying the medical treatment may be what is important, rather than the treatment itself.) More research is needed into both the effectiveness and safety of hormonal supplementation (see also p. 105).

Other possible causes

Mother's age

The risk of spontaneous miscarriage does appear to increase slightly with age, most obviously so after 30, whether or not the fetus is chromosomally normal. Older women are more likely to miscarry both abnormal and normal fetuses, but it must be remembered that most older mothers do have successful pregnancies and that the prospects are very good.

Father's age

Most attention in the past has focused on the mother, not the father, so there is little evidence to show whether paternal age may play a part in producing a risk of miscarriage. One study, however, does seem to show that there is an association between increased paternal age and an increased rate of miscarriage which is stronger than the association with increased maternal age, although other studies have yet to confirm this finding. It is possible, of course, that with older fathers, intercourse may be less frequent and the sperm will therefore be older and perhaps more prone to abnormality, leading to an increased risk of miscarriage, but more investigation is needed before any firm conclusions can be drawn. On the other hand, immature sperm are also thought to be a possible cause of abnormality, and this situation is most likely to occur when lovemaking is very frequent, so it would seem that ideally couples should pace their lovemaking to ensure that the sperm are mature but not too mature –a practical suggestion, maybe, but not exactly a very romantic or spontaneous one!

Psychological factors and stress

When no other causes can be found, doctors are sometimes tempted to look for a psychosomatic cause but there is little evidence to support this suggestion. There is, however, evidence which suggests that good emotional support may have a positive effect in promoting a successful pregnancy. Studies exist which suggest that a stressed animal is more likely to miscarry and therefore it is possible that this could apply to human mothers-to-be as well. Naturally, it is not always possible to avoid stress during pregnancy because unexpected events can be imposed on us at any time, but where possible it would seem sensible to avoid known sources of stress and to set aside time for you and your baby to relax (see p. 110 for further details).

Smoking, alcohol and drugs

These are all forms of stress imposed on the developing fetus. If you are addicted and unable to cope without intake of one or more of the above, then forgive me for not pulling my punches because I do appreciate how difficult it would be for you to abstain, but this is one area where the evidence is now irrefutable – smoking, drinking alcohol or taking drugs increases the risk of damage to your growing baby and increases the risk of miscarriage. The anxious time of pregnancy is not the ideal time to try and give up something which has a powerful hold on you, but if you have suffered a miscarriage, it would be well worth trying to reduce or stop your intake before embarking on another pregnancy, to give your next baby the best possible chance of survival. Support is available, so it is worth giving some thought to contacting those who could help you.

It is not just mothers-to-be who bear a responsibility. The possible effects of male drinking and smoking on sperm quality and subsequent miscarriage have not yet been sufficiently studied but it is known that men who drink heavily have more abnormal sperm, as do men who smoke heavily. Although the reproductive effect of smoking in men has not yet been properly studied, there are suggestions that smoking impairs fertility and certainly reduces the birth weight of babies. Organizations such as Foresight therefore emphasize the need to promote good preconceptual care in both mothers *and* fathers and this is worth bearing in mind.

Sexual intercourse and internal examinations

There is no evidence to suggest that lovemaking during pregnancy can cause miscarriage. For those of us who are pregnant, some doctors advise avoiding intercourse during the first three months at the times when our period would have been due, and also at the times of previous miscarriages. For peace of mind it would seem sensible to follow our doctors' advice, but otherwise we're allowed to go ahead and enjoy ourselves!

Some women do worry about the possible effect of an internal examination during early pregnancy, especially if this is followed soon afterwards by a miscarriage. But miscarriages do happen most frequently during early pregnancy and therefore the likelihood is that the association is purely one of chance, resulting from the stage of pregnancy involved. There is no evidence to suggest that an internal examination can cause miscarriage, but if you would prefer not to have one, you are entitled to say so.

Illness

If you are ill during early pregnancy and then have a miscarriage it is tempting to blame the illness as the cause. There is little evidence to support this, except when there has been high fever, but on the other hand some infections and illnesses *are* known to play a part in miscarriage.

Listeriosis

Listeria is a bacteria which, unlike others, can multiply at fridge temperatures. It is capable of contaminating some ready-cooked chilled meals and some soft cheeses, and so pregnant women are advised to avoid such meals and to avoid eating cheeses such as brie, camembert and blue-vein varieties (hard cheeses, cheese spreads and processed cottage cheeses are *not* a risk). If you would like further information and advice, the address and telephone number of the Listeria Society are listed at the end of the book.

Rubella (German measles)

The results of catching rubella in early pregnancy can be tragic. Even if you do not miscarry, your baby may suffer severe damage, so every woman should check that she is immune to rubella before becoming pregnant. Even if you have had German measles as a child or received immunization at school, your immunity level can fall in later years. A quick blood test before pregnancy will give you peace of mind and allow you to proceed safe in the knowledge that any resulting baby will be protected.

Mycoplasma and ureaplasma

These infections are neither viruses nor bacteria but they are like viruses and can exist in the cervix or uterus. They can be responsible for non-specific urethritis and they are associated with miscarriage. They can be identified by culturing tissue from the cervix and uterus and can be treated before pregnancy with one of the tetracycline drugs. It is wise to treat your partner at the same time, to avoid the risk of cross-infection.

Cytomegalovirus, toxoplasma, brucella and chlamydia

Like mycoplasma, these are thought to be implicated as possible causes of miscarriage. Cytomegalovirus (CMV) is a virus which gives a 'flu-like illness, usually with swollen glands. Toxoplasmosis can be caught as a result of eating raw meat (which is still rare in this country!) or by coming into contact with the infected faeces of cats. Anyone who owns a cat or has neighbouring cats who use their garden should therefore take extra care if they are pregnant or hoping to be so and should use rubber gloves when emptying litter trays or working in the garden. (For anyone wanting further information or advice, the address and telephone number of the Toxoplasmosis Trust are given at the end of the book.) Brucellosis is a bacterial infection known to cause abortion in farm animals but not conclusively proven as a cause of miscarriage in humans. Similarly, the organism *chlamydia psittaci* is known to cause spontaneous abortion in sheep and therefore as a safeguard, pregnant women are advised to avoid involvement with lambing or any material relating to lambing, and if their partners are involved, they are advised to take extra care with general hygiene.

Herpes and syphilis

Known to be two extremely unpleasant infections and thankfully not too common, but again you should ensure that any possibility of infection with either of these viruses is thoroughly investigated and treated before embarking on a pregnancy, as they are known to affect the developing baby.

AIDS

It is not yet known whether infection with the HIV (human immunosuppressive virus which can lead to AIDS) could increase the risk of miscarriage but it is known that it can be transmitted to the baby during pregnancy and it is therefore very important for anyone who thinks that she could be carrying the HIV to have a blood test before trying to become pregnant.

Diabetes, thyroid problems, kidney disease, high blood pressure

Certain illnesses such as these may lead to complications in pregnancy but there is little evidence to show whether they are implicated in miscarriage and the current view is that they are rarely significant as a possible cause.

Immunological causes

In a sense the developing fetus is a 'foreign body' in that half of the chromosomes come from the father and therefore one might expect the mother's immune system to activate and try to reject the fetus just as it would any other foreign body (such as bacteria). Obviously some system operates during pregnancy to prevent this from happening and it is thought that the mother needs to 'recognize' the fetus as foreign first in order for this special pregnancy response to be activated. If the chromosomes of the mother and father are too similar and as a result they have similar HLA (human lymphocytic antigens) tissue types, it seems possible that the mother's body may fail to recognize the fetus as foreign and will therefore not activate the special immune response which protects the fetus from rejection. If this is thought to be the case and to be causing recurrent miscarriage, treatment is sometimes available in the form of a transfusion of white blood cells which stimulates the production of antibodies, thereby boosting the mother's immune system and increasing the chances of her body recognizing the fetus as foreign and triggering the protective pregnancy immune response. In some cases the blood cells may come from the partner, in others they may come from other donors, and are usually given just before conception or during the first eight weeks of pregnancy. Some centres are reporting good success rates, but there have also been reports of a higher incidence of premature and small-for-dates babies and an increased risk of stillbirth or neonatal death. If you feel that an immunological problem may be relevent in your case it is worth enquiring about the possibility of treatment, although you would need to weigh up all the existing evidence before deciding whether to try and proceed.

Environmental factors

Environmental factors such as lead (at your work place or if you live near a lead smelter), toxic chemicals and irradiation have been cited as possible causes of miscarriage. Some of these toxins cannot be avoided, but it would make sense to avoid contact with X-rays during pregnancy if at all possible. Even if you do not think you are pregnant, it is worth bearing in mind the 'Ten-day Rule', namely, to avoid the ten days preceding your next expected period just in case you may be about to ovulate, or may, unknown to yourself, have just conceived.

Occupation

As you no doubt know, if your work brings you into contact with radiation, then you should ask for and use protective screening. Nurses who assist in theatre in any way should also be aware of the potential risk posed by unintentionally inhaling anaesthetic being administered to patients during surgical operations. If your work involves using a visual display unit (VDU), then it is worth trying to find out the latest results of studies. Concern that working with VDUs may cause miscarriage has prompted a number of studies, but so far the results are mixed. Three major investigations concluded that VDUs are probably safe to use during pregnancy, but an American study in 1988 showed an increased risk of miscarriage. If you would like to find out more, there is an address at the end of this book to which you could write. If you are unhappy about using a VDU while you are pregnant, ask for redeployment away from the screen, or at least take hourly breaks, if only for your own peace of mind.

Diet

Certain foods, or the lack of them, have been linked at various times with miscarriage, but the evidence is inconclusive. One factor that does seem to be relevant, however, is deficiency of the B vitamin folic acid, found in green vegetables, salads and liver. As part of ensuring that you are as healthy as possible before trying to conceive, a suitable intake (via a supplement if necessary) would therefore seem sensible (see p. 107 for further details of preconceptual care).

Contraception

Most couples nowadays try to plan their children and use some form of contraception until they are ready to start a family.

The Pill

There is no existing evidence to suggest that using the Pill prior to conception increases the risk of miscarriage; in fact one study suggests a decreased risk. There is, however, some suggestion that becoming pregnant while on the Pill may slightly increase the risk of miscarriage. After an ectopic pregnancy (a pregnancy that takes place outside the uterus (e.g. in the Fallopian tubes) (see p. 28) use of the progesterone-only Pill has been linked with an increased risk of having another ectopic pregnancy.

IUD (Intrauterine (contraceptive) device)

Use of the IUD – the 'coil' – has also been linked with an increased risk of having an ectopic pregnancy because the coil prevents the fertilized egg from implanting in the uterus and thereby increases the possibility of it implanting elsewhere. Some pregnancies (between 1 per cent and 3 per cent) do occur while the coil is still in the uterus. When this happens there is an increased risk of bleeding and miscarriage, and of complications, together with an increased risk of infection. If you discover that you are pregnant, then it is best to see your doctor and have the IUD removed as soon as possible, but if the strings are not visible then the coil is best left alone. Even removing the coil incurs a risk of miscarriage, but it is less than the risk involved if the coil is left (which may be as high as 50 per cent). On a more positive note, many pregnancies resulting from IUD failure do continue without problems, but the potential risks of using an IUD should be borne in mind when choosing which form of contraception to use.

Barrier methods

Condoms for men and diaphragms for women, used with or without spermicides, are widely used methods of contraception and do not have any known effect on miscarriage rates.

Previous miscarriages, induced abortions or dilation and curettage operations

Evidence suggests that a single induced abortion is most unlikely to increase the risk of subsequent miscarriage. This is also true for a dilation and curettage ('D and C' or 'scrape') operation (unless it was performed prior to 1973, when the methods used to dilate the cervix instrumentally sometimes caused damage, leading to future complications such as cervical incompetence). It is thought that fewer than 4 per cent of miscarriages can be attributed to previous induced abortion, which should reassure anyone worrying that her previous induced abortion may have caused her subsequent miscarriage. Having a previous miscarriage does slightly increase the risk of having another, but the statistics are still very encouraging, with a 76 per cent chance of having a successful pregnancy (74 per cent after two miscarriages and 68 per cent after three or more).

Accidents

If an accident, such as a fall, is followed by a miscarriage it is very tempting to blame it as the cause. Indeed, in a survey carried out in 1983, 11 per cent of women interviewed named an accident, illness or medication as the cause of their miscarriage; in a survey back in 1819 as many as 35 per cent of women who had miscarried named accidents, illness or medication. Perhaps this is an indication that in the absence of other identifiable causes, we search around for our own fated contribution. There is no scientific evidence, however, to suggest that accidental injury to the abdomen causes miscarriage, except in the rare case of severe injury following, for example, a car crash. Although minor injury should not, of itself, cause miscarriage, the trauma surrounding it may play a part – if, for example, a woman has suffered the deeply distressing experience of being knocked about by her partner during pregnancy. It is also possible that stress in other forms may be a relevant factor (see pp. 8 and 109–10).

Lifting and physical strain

This is a possible cause which is often suggested by women who experience miscarriage but which appears to have no scientific evidence to support it. Women who move house during pregnancy very often blame themselves afterwards if miscarriage subsequently takes place, believing that they have caused the miscarriage because of all the heavy lifting and physical strain involved. Despite being assured to the contrary, I am still tempted to blame heavy lifting for my own early miscarriage, so I am no exception and although there really does not seem to be any valid basis for such a belief, it is difficult to dismiss the instinctive feeling that strenuous lifting or straining prior to a miscarriage must somehow have played a part.

Miscarriage after ultrasound, chorionic villus sampling, amniocentesis, fetoscopy or cordocentesis

So far there is no evidence to suggest any association between the use of ultrasound (see p. 26 for further details) and miscarriage. However, there is *animal* evidence of ultrasound damage and no one yet knows the possible dangers of passing high-energy sound waves through a vulnerable developing fetus. On the other hand, ultrasound can be extremely useful in the diagnosis of possible pregnancy complications and of threatened miscarriage. One of the occasions when ultrasound is invaluable is in the accurate locating of the fetus and placenta prior to chorionic villus sampling (CVS), amniocentesis, fetoscopy or cordoscopy – all are techniques used to diagnose abnormalities in the developing baby which occasionally precipitate a miscarriage (for further details of these techniques, see p. 104). Unfortunately all these techniques do carry a slight risk of miscarriage, the least being cordocentesis as this is the least invasive. If there is reason to suspect a neural tube malformation (such as spina bifida or anencephaly) a test does now exist known as the alphafetoprotein test. This involves a simple blood test for a substance known as alphafetoprotein, which if present in the mother's blood in high amounts acts as an indication of fetal abnormalities. This test does not carry the potential risk associated with the other techniques and the normal level of alphafetoprotein can be very reassuring, but obviously if the blood test indicates that an abnormality could be present then further tests would have to be conducted, with their own attendant slight risk of miscarriage and the heartrending need to decide whether or not to terminate the pregnancy if an abnormality is confirmed.

Tests, investigations and treatments

These important topics will be discussed in Chapter 8, to help those who are considering whether to risk trying to have another baby.

From everything that has been said in this opening chapter, it is clear that much more research is needed, together with correctly controlled and fully evaluated studies. Yes, miscarriage is a common and some would say trivial medical event, but it can be profoundly traumatic to the woman experiencing it and its potential physical and emotional effects should never be underestimated.

2

The Physical Impact

Every woman's experience of miscarriage is unique to herself. Women who have suffered recurrent miscarriage have told me that each one has been very different. It is not just the range in time that can vary so much – from so early on that the pregnancy has barely been confirmed to so late that the life of the baby is almost viable – it is also the range in physical symptoms and sensations before, during and after the miscarriage itself. In this chapter I would like to focus on the physical impact of miscarriage and on how much it can vary, because so often what is perceived by medical staff does not in any way correspond to what is being perceived and felt by the mother who is losing her baby.

Definitions

Three sets of definitions need to be given before continuing any further, and I'm sorry if these seem yet more cold facts to take on board, but it helps to know the meaning of the terms which tend to be used by medical professionals at the time of the miscarriage.

Embryo and fetus
The first set of definitions concerns the baby. What to most of us is a real baby growing inside us – until the harsh reality of the miscarriage – is viewed medically in a much more detached and clinical way. From weeks 2 to 8 of gestation (i.e. pregnancy) the fertilized ovum is regarded as an embryo. From 9 weeks until birth the embryo becomes regarded as a fetus. The mother who was greeted at each antenatal visit with: 'And how's baby coming along?' will soon find after miscarriage that this same baby apparently never existed, that her loss was merely that of a 'fetus'. Reducing the status of the baby in this way may help the medical staff to cope with the situation, but it does little to comfort the bereaved mother whose awareness of the nature of her loss is only too real.

Miscarriage and stillbirth
At the moment, a miscarriage up to 28 weeks of pregnancy is

regarded as that of a fetus, not a baby, and a dead fetus has no legal status, is not registered as a birth or a death and is not granted a recognized burial. From 28 weeks onwards, if the baby is born and shows no sign of life, the event ceases to be regarded as a miscarriage and becomes known as a stillbirth. The baby's birth and death have to be registered and a burial arranged. Clearly the medical and legal definitions are currently at odds with developments in obstetric and paediatric services, for many babies born before 28 weeks do now survive. Because of such progress, in 1988 the Stillbirth and Neonatal Death Society, supported by the Miscarriage Association, the National Childbirth Trust and many professionals in nursing, midwifery, general practice and obstetrics, wrote to the Secretary of State for Health asking for the legal definition of stillbirth to be lowered to 24 weeks' gestation. The subject was raised in a debate in the House of Commons on 5 February 1991, but an outcome is still awaited.

Types of miscarriage

The third set of definitions concerns the terms used medically to describe the different types of miscarriage which can occur. Again, these terms are sometimes totally at odds with what the mother is feeling and experiencing. The medical profession tends to use the term 'abortion' although we use the term 'miscarriage' for what we experience. Whilst deliberate abortion is not undergone lightly, to use the term 'abortion' for miscarriage is very regrettable because it has such painful connotations for anyone suffering the loss of a much-wanted baby. After my late miscarriage I had to have a D and C operation nine weeks later and I can still remember how distressed I felt to see the word 'abortion' on my hospital form. It would be very helpful if the medical profession could show some sensitivity by agreeing to adapt their terminology to meet the needs of mothers, bringing 'miscarriage' into general use and reserving the term 'abortion' solely for the active termination of a pregnancy.

Blighted ovum (or anembryonic pregnancy)

It is thought that up to 60 per cent of all miscarriages are the result of 'blighted ova' where the placenta and membranes form but there is no baby because the fertilized ovum is poorly developed or has not developed at all. An ultrasound scan will reveal that there is a placenta and sac but no baby, even though the woman feels pregnant. Usually such a pregnancy miscarries between 6–10 weeks, but sometimes everything simply shrinks inside and no miscarriage takes place, giving rise to the situation known as 'missed abortion' (see below).

Spontaneous abortion

This is the medical term for what we know as miscarriage and at present it means the expulsion of a fetus from the uterus before 28 weeks of pregnancy.

Induced abortion

This has nothing to do with miscarriage and means the deliberate termination of a pregnancy.

Threatened abortion

This indicates that the pregnancy may be in danger, the most usual sign being spotting or bleeding from the vagina, sometimes accompanied by a slight cramping type of pain. At this stage it is often impossible to know whether the bleeding has any significance, since many women who experience early bleeding go on to have normal pregnancies and healthy, full-term babies.

Inevitable abortion

If the bleeding increases and the pain becomes severe, loss of the baby is usually inevitable and once the neck of the uterus (known as the cervix) opens, nothing can be done to prevent the fetus from being expelled.

Incomplete abortion

This is the term used when miscarriage takes place but some of the contents of the uterus (known medically as 'products of conception') remain behind, leading to continued symptoms of miscarriage including bleeding. It is a serious condition and surgical intervention may be required to prevent haemorrhage and infection.

Complete abortion

This means that when the miscarriage takes place, the fetus, amniotic sac and placenta come away completely, with nothing left behind.

Missed abortion

It sometimes happens that the fetus dies or fails to develop properly but is not immediately expelled by the mother's body. This can be very confusing for the mother since the obvious signs of pregnancy tend to subside and there may be some spotting of blood and yet the mother knows that miscarriage has not occurred. Sometimes spontaneous miscarriage takes place at a later date, but if this does not happen then it is necessary to have the contents of the womb removed either by a process known as vacuum aspiration or by an operation known as a 'D and C' (dilation – or dilatation – and curettage). Nowadays it is less likely for women to endure long delays as ultrasound scans are able to determine whether a missed abortion has occurred and if this is the case, appropriate surgical action can then be taken.

Habitual abortion/recurrent abortion

This is the term used when miscarriage occurs during three or more consecutive pregnancies.

Septic abortion

This is the term used when an infection of the uterus follows a miscarriage or abortion. It is most likely to occur when the miscarriage has been incomplete, hence the need on occasions for a D and C operation to try and prevent the risk of infection from arising.

How do I know if I'm miscarrying?

When we become pregnant for the first time, it is all new to us, each sign and stage of pregnancy is a revelation, a voyage where some of the discoveries are definitely more pleasant than others. Our bodies seem to become in some ways entirely independent of us and beyond our control. Nobody willingly opts in the early stages for morning sickness, nor in the later stages for heartburn, cramps and a totally unreliable bladder, but because it is all part of a positive process we are able to surrender ourselves to the new and dominant role which our bodies are playing – and never more so than during labour when no matter how much we might wish to delay, when our bodies say push, we push! The same is true of miscarriage. The first time it happens to us it is all new and we don't know what to expect, but with this particular voyage it is a totally negative process and consequently a very frightening one. Our body is beyond our control, as in labour, but although we know that there can be no happy outcome we are powerless to prevent the process and this can make us feel completely at odds with our own body and somehow deeply betrayed.

Sometimes the miscarriage happens quickly, but at other times it can be a long drawn-out process, with symptoms coming and going, and this can be very confusing and distressing for the mother concerned. Not surprisingly she can feel in a form of limbo, with her hopes alternately being raised or dashed depending on the symptoms which she is experiencing. Despite the evidence of physical indications that a miscarriage is threatening, she is likely to go on hoping against hope that all will be well, fighting her own body to try and retain the baby. At such times there is likely to be a strong feeling of helplessness. Once the miscarriage becomes inevitable it can almost be a relief because it ends the time of limbo and allows action to take place.

Symptoms of miscarriage

Bleeding
This is often the first and most common sign that something may be wrong, but the nature and amount of bleeding can vary greatly. It must be remembered that bleeding in early pregnancy does not necessarily mean that a miscarriage will follow and if the bleeding stops and the baby is carried to term, then it is as likely as any other baby to be completely normal. Studies suggest that anywhere between 1 in 100 and 20 or more in 100 pregnancies may show some early bleeding (the rate depending to some extent on the definition of bleeding and the methods of reporting it). In early pregnancy, this may simply be a partially suppressed period, happening because the body has not made enough pregnancy hormones to stop the period completely.

Most bleeding in early pregnancy comes from inside the uterus where the placenta is attaching itself to the wall of the uterus, but other less common causes do exist, such as an erosion (destruction of the surface layer of tissue due to injury or infection) or polyp (a swelling or protrusion) of the cervix or lesions in the vagina. Bleeding as a sign of impending miscarriage can vary between slight spotting, a brown discharge or loss of fresh blood which may be slight or copious. The bleeding may keep stopping and starting and there may be only a mild loss, or the bleeding may become very heavy and this can be very frightening, especially if the mother is at home on her own and may genuinely fear that she may haemorrhage and die before being found. Even if she is able to make her way to a hospital casualty department, the situation can be very distressing. Her expectation is that her needs will be immediately met, but the reality is more often that she will be kept waiting on a stretcher or a hard hospital chair, afraid not only of what is happening to her but also of the potentially acute embarrassment of flooding the chair and floor in full public view. A society that still finds it difficult to acknowledge openly that women menstruate is certainly not ready to cope with the sight of the profuse blood loss which can accompany a miscarriage and the risk of this happening simply adds to the distress which the mother is already feeling.

Occasionally, especially if the miscarriage is incomplete, heavy bleeding can become a medical emergency. Ergometrine or Syntocinon injections can help to limit the bleeding, but some women may find themselves needing an intravenous drip or blood transfusion and this may have to be accompanied by manual removal of the contents of the uterus, or an ERPC (evacuation of the retained products of conception) or a D and C operation.

Pain, contractions or backache

Some women experience period-type pains, others pain in the stomach or thighs and yet others a type of low backache which may range from mild to severe. Again, of course, all these symptoms can occur during pregnancy and do not necessarily mean that a miscarriage is inevitable, but they should not be ignored, especially if they are accompanied by any form of bleeding.

Absence of symptoms

Sometimes there are no symptoms at all and the first indication that the pregnancy is not going to remain viable is revealed at a routine antenatal scan. This usually means that there has been a blighted ovum (see p. 18) or a missed abortion (see p. 19) and the shock of such a discovery is even greater than when instinct has forewarned the mother that something is wrong. It can seem very unreal to go for a routine antenatal session feeling pregnant and happy and normal, only to discover that there is no baby at all or that the baby has already died.

Other symptoms

Many women describe having 'flu-like symptoms before a

miscarriage, or simply a feeling of being somehow unwell. Others describe a foreboding or an intuitive feeling that something is wrong. Of course, some people will argue that most women have times of uneasiness during pregnancy and that these tend to be forgotten if the pregnancy progresses and only remembered if it ceases to be viable. However, intuition should never be dismissed on such grounds since that does not alter the fact that a woman's intuition often can be right.

Reduction in signs of pregnancy

With early threatened miscarriage, some women notice that their breasts are no longer so tender or 'tingly' or that their morning sickness has ceased. With later threatened miscarriage they may notice that their abdomen is no longer enlarging.

Often women experiencing their first pregnancy are reluctant to report observations such as reduction in pregnancy signs for fear of being seen as making a fuss or being regarded as neurotic. This tends to be true where other symptoms such as pain or bleeding are concerned as well, and after the miscarriage occurs many women then feel guilty for not seeking medical aid sooner. But the stark reality is that very often nothing can be done to prevent miscarriage from taking place; doctors can offer much in the way of support but little in the way of prevention, no matter how much they would like to do so. Even the time-honoured practice of recommending bed-rest remains unproven as a preventive measure.

What happens during a miscarriage?

Some women cope alone at home when they know they are miscarrying, but most (over 90 per cent according to one survey) contact their doctor. The response of their doctor can vary greatly, from nothing more than telephoned advice to rest, to a home visit or arranged admission to hospital. Of those in the survey who contacted their doctor, over 75 per cent were admitted to hospital and nearly all these later underwent an ERPC or D and C operation (see p. 27 for further details).

Some doctors prefer to recommend bed-rest before making any decision regarding hospital admission, in the hope that the pregnancy will 'settle down' and the risk of miscarriage pass of its own accord. Sometimes such hopes are realized, but if the symptoms · continue or increase then hospital admission is usually arranged unless the mother opts to remain at home. Being in hospital should have the advantage of access to immediate medical reassurance and care should the need arise (such as a blood transfusion or a D and C). Being at home has the advantage of privacy in familiar surroundings, with the least disruption to family routine.

Early miscarriage

Sometimes the mother has no choice but to be at home, if the actual miscarriage happens very rapidly. That is exactly what happened to me when I experienced a very early miscarriage at about 8 weeks. I had spent the previous Friday evening helping friends to carry great sackloads of jumble out of cars, along a main street and down a long alleyway to a church hall in readiness for a charity jumble sale the next morning. When I got home that night, exhausted, I found that I was bleeding. The elation I had been feeling all that week at knowing that I was pregnant immediately turned to panic at the thought that I might miscarry, but with an effort I pushed aside my fears. The following morning the bleeding had stopped, so I went ahead with helping at the jumble sale because they were short-staffed, but did my best to rest for the remainder of the weekend. During that time the bleeding kept starting and stopping again, but by the Monday morning I felt unwell with severe low back pain, so instead of going to work (I was a playgroup supervisor at the time) I arranged a replacement and stayed at home. The back pain continued but it was not until mid-morning that I realized that, even at the very early stage of 8 weeks, I was in a form of full labour. Feeling a sudden urgent need for the toilet, I went to our outside one as it was the nearest. By then it was too late to summon help and I could not have done so anyway. I had not realized that early miscarriage could involve true contractions and labour and sat watching in an amazed and almost detached way as my body went through the final stages, culminating in the passing of a copious amount of blood which included a number of very large clots. There was something unreal about the whole episode. 'So that's it, then' I thought, flushed the toilet and returned to the kitchen.

The physical impact was brief. The emotional impact took much longer to acknowledge and work through, for having experienced a brief but genuine labour I can now see that I later experienced an equally genuine postnatal depression as my poor confused hormones tried to sort themselves out. Irrationally, but perhaps understandably to anyone who has experienced miscarriage at home, I was greatly relieved the following year when we extended our kitchen and removed the outside toilet in the process. From the day of the miscarriage I had relegated it to a storage room, never wanting to be in it again.

Because mine was such an early miscarriage I saw only clots. Many women undergoing a later miscarriage pass a recognizable embryo or fetus, their own tiny but usually perfect baby. This can be an incredible shock and can leave the mother totally bewildered as to what to do. To simply flush the tiny body away down the toilet seems callous in the extreme and somehow obscene, but to retrieve and take it to hospital for investigation can seem equally obscene and almost a betrayal. If an open fire is available at home, then cremation becomes a possibility. If a garden at home is available, then a private garden burial is often the most satisfying solution to a deeply distressing problem.

Ironically, for those who are able to steel themselves to take the embryo or fetus to hospital, the action is often a waste of time. Investigations are not usually carried out until at least three consecutive miscarriages have occurred and even then, what can be done in the way of investigating a miscarried embryo or fetus is at present very limited. If the fetus is available, it will usually be examined for any obvious abnormalities. In the absence of a fetus, any tissue available should be examined firstly to confirm that the bleeding was because of a pregnancy and not because of any other cause and secondly to exclude the possibility of a 'molar' pregnancy (see p. 31). Other tests, however, are not usually done because of a number of reasons; (1) limited resources (2) the fact that little is likely to be discovered (3) the fact that tests for infection or chromosomal abnormalities are complicated, expensive, time-consuming and not necessarily productive (4) the fact that certain tests can only be conducted on fresh tissue and (5) the medical recognition that miscarriage is often a one-off, self-righting event usually followed by a successful pregnancy.

What the doctor may do

Naturally the stage of pregnancy at which miscarriage occurs will influence the nature of the miscarriage and the medical response. Whereas some doctors advocate bed-rest and non-interference if miscarriage appears to be threatening at an early stage of pregnancy, others prefer to conduct an internal examination to determine whether the cervix is closed or open (once the cervix thins and opens, miscarriage becomes inevitable). He or she may also carry out a pregnancy test, check for the baby's heartbeat or arrange for the hospital to do so, using a Sonicaid fetal heart detector if pregnancy has reached the appropriate stage, or he or she may arrange for an ultrasound scan. The use of scans has reduced the need for internal examinations, so if you would prefer not to have such an examination or feel that it might increase the risk of miscarriage, you are entitled to ask your doctor to postpone it in the hope that it will prove not to be necessary.

Ultrasound works by passing high-frequency, short-wavelength sound waves through the uterus and its contents. The waves pass easily through fluid but bounce back off the solid surfaces of the fetus and the placenta and the resulting pattern of reflected sound is then translated and projected onto a form of television screen, producing pictures which can be photographed. After about 8 weeks of pregnancy, the heartbeat can actually be seen. Ultrasound scanning works on the same principle which enables submarines to navigate or bats to fly at night and it can give important information about the absence or presence of a fetus, including size and position. Scanning is not foolproof, however, for sometimes the pregnancy sac may be poorly visualized or even obscured, and as yet no one can be certain about possible dangers involved in passing high-energy sound waves through a vulnerable developing fetus. Existing knowledge indicates that scans are safe, but then for many years X-rays during pregnancy were also considered to be safe until this was found to be untrue, so any mother offered the opportunity of an ultrasound scan will need to weigh up the pros and cons before giving her consent.

If pregnancy tests are carried out, these will indicate the presence or absence of HCG, human chorionic gonadotrophin, a hormone found in the urine of pregnant women. Unfortunately they are not totally reliable because it can take several days for HCG to be cleared from the body and therefore the tests can continue to give positive readings for a while even though the mother may already have miscarried or the baby already be dead. Often it is a combination of investigations which will enable a doctor to say with any certainty whether a miscarriage has occurred or will occur in the near future.

Operations

Sometimes early miscarriages are complete at the time and the mother's body is able to recover quite quickly, but at other times these miscarriages prove to be incomplete, and then there is a risk of infection and/or severe bleeding. Between 6 and 16 weeks of pregnancy it can be difficult to tell whether the miscarriage has been complete and scans cannot always give an accurate assessment, so doctors often recommend manual removal, an ERPC (evacuation of retained products of conception) or a D and C (dilation and curettage), which means that, under anaesthetic, the cervix is dilated and the lining of the uterus gently scraped to remove any remaining products of pregnancy. Some doctors prefer to advise waiting and monitoring the bleeding for a few days following a miscarriage, to give the mother's body a chance to right itself without the need for medical intervention, but others prefer to arrange an operation as soon as possible, to minimize the risk of infection or heavy bleeding. If a miscarriage has not occurred but a scan shows beyond doubt that there is just an empty sac or that the fetus is dead, then most doctors would advocate an immediate D and C.

Reactions to the need for an ERPC or D & C can vary and these will be discussed in Chapter 7, but it is important when considering the impact of an ERPC or D and C to know that these remain a very common medical response to the event of miscarriage.

Late miscarriage

Miscarriages which occur after 16 weeks are much less common, but labour during mid-term pregnancy can be very painful and difficult because the mother is so unprepared both physically and emotionally. After 16 weeks an ERPC is not possible because of the size of the fetus; a D and C remains an option, but only if the doctor is convinced that the baby is dead. Otherwise, labour has to be experienced, either naturally or induced by means of synthetic hormones via a drip or pessaries. The later the stage of pregnancy at which miscarriage occurs, the more like a true birth it will seem. Those who miscarry from 19 weeks onwards (and sometimes sooner) are likely to produce milk afterwards, between two and five days following the miscarriage. This can be very distressing emotionally as it reinforces the loss of the baby, and very distressing physically as the breasts can become engorged and painful. The best advice seems to be to take painkillers (such as paracetamol) if necessary and to reduce fluid intake to a minimum for a few days, leaving the breasts alone as much as possible and only expressing the milk if absolutely necessary, since expressing will tend to encourage more milk to come. Homeopathic remedies are available and it might be worth enquiring about these. Some medical professionals still advise binding the breasts to encourage suppression of milk. Alternatively some doctors may prescribe medication such as Parlodel or Estrovis to dry up the milk, but there are mixed views about whether it is wise to do so because of possible side-effects and most prefer to allow the milk to wane of its own accord.

Ectopic pregnancy and hydatidiform mole

Thankfully both of these conditions are relatively rare, but they warrant a section to themselves because not only do they carry the trauma and loss which accompany miscarriage, they also carry possible implications for future pregnancies.

Ectopic pregnancy

Ectopic pregnancy (derived from the Greek word *ektopos* meaning one that is 'out of place') is one which develops outside the uterus. The most likely site for ectopic embedding is in one of the Fallopian tubes. This is as likely in one tube as in the other, and occurs probably in over 90 per cent of all ectopic pregnancies, although embedding can also take place where the tube joins the uterus (known as cornual), at the site of one of the ovaries (ovarian), or in the abdominal cavity or elsewhere. In virtually all cases the outlook is bleak because the embryo, if it survives and continues to develop and expand, will eventually cause a rupture which can become a life-threatening event to the mother because of the sudden and severe bleeding which may result. Because of this it is very important that ectopic pregnancy is diagnosed and treated as soon as possible and it is therefore essential for women to know the likely symptoms so that they can seek medical help without delay.

Ectopic pregnancy is on the increase, not just in the UK but also in other countries such as the USA, Finland, Sweden and Czechoslovakia. In 1966 the estimate for England and Wales was 3.2 per 1000 conceptions. By 1976 this had risen to 5 per 1000; by 1990 the figure had doubled. More ectopic pregnancies are now discovered at early scans that might previously have miscarried before being recorded; nevertheless it is a disturbing trend. The two possible causes most frequently cited are pelvic infection and use of the coil (IUD). Infection is cited as a cause because of damage to the normal function of the tube (namely to transport the fertilized ovum safely to the uterus), and the coil, because its prevention of intrauterine implantation may increase the risk of implantation taking place elsewhere. Certainly users of the IUD are known to be at higher risk of ectopic pregnancy (some say about 6 times greater than in the general population, others about 10 times greater). The use of the progestogen-only contraceptive pill has also been cited, along with other possible causes, but as yet such theories lack accurate supporting evidence and more investigation is needed to refute or substantiate them.

Pain and bleeding are the two most common symptoms, the pain often occurring on one distinct side of the abdomen and frequently accompanied by a feeling of faintness. In about two-thirds of all cases one or two periods will have been missed and the normal signs of pregnancy will be present. The problem is that these symptoms can accompany the threatened miscarriage of a uterine pregnancy as well and it is therefore quite easy for ectopic pregnancy to remain undiagnosed until it has become a medical emergency, especially since the severe pain associated with it can be confused with appendicitis. Occasionally the pressure of internal bleeding in the abdominal cavity can result in referred pain occurring in the tip of the shoulder and this can aid accurate diagnosis, but this only happens in about 1 per cent of cases.

When the fertilized egg implants in one of the Fallopian tubes, many of the symptoms of normal early pregnancy still result. The pregnancy hormone HCG is produced, the uterus begins to enlarge, the breasts become tender, the next period is missed and a urine pregnancy test may prove positive (this positive result happens in approximately half of all ectopic pregnancies, but a more recent test known as the radioimmunoassay test is more accurate and can even on occasions distinguish ruptured from unruptured ectopic pregnancies).

In about a third of all ectopic pregnancies, rupture of the tube takes place and this usually occurs between the 8th and 12th week (depending on whether the pregnancy is in the narrower or the broader end of the tube). It causes acute pain and bleeding which may be sudden and severe enough to cause the woman to collapse, although more often the tubal rupture is a gradual process, with intermittent vaginal bleeding and pain. When the tube ruptures, the embryo dies and is reabsorbed into the mother's body just as it would be in other mammals. Usually the symptoms of pregnancy will then recede and pregnancy tests will prove negative.

If the doctor suspects an ectopic pregnancy, for safety's sake he or she usually arranges for hospital admission and may arrange for a laparoscopy to be done (in which the inside of the pelvis is viewed with a fine instrument inserted through an inch-wide slit in the navel). If this confirms the ectopic pregnancy, it will be followed by a laparotomy, an incision in the lower abdomen to remove the tubal pregnancy. Often rupture takes place before either course of action can be carried out although occasionally, if the ectopic pregnancy is diagnosed early enough, it is sometimes possible to 'milk out' the pregnancy from the tube, leaving the tube undamaged but ending the pregnancy as it is not possible to transfer it to the uterus. More often, sadly, it is necessary to remove the tube by means of an operation (a 'salpingectomy'). Sometimes the ovary linked to the tube has to be removed as well (a salpingo–oophorectomy; when this happens, the remaining ovary 'doubles up' its function and ovulation occurs each month from the one ovary).

Those are the bare facts, but they do nothing in the way of conveying the pain and trauma which accompany ectopic pregnancy, with the added distress of knowing that not only has the pregnancy which should have led to a baby been lost but also that the chances of having a future baby have been reduced, together with the ever-present fear that ectopic pregnancy could happen again.

After surgery for ectopic pregnancy, the woman will need time to recover from the effects of the anaesthetic and the operation itself. There will be pain from the wound and exhaustion from the shock and the blood loss. If the blood loss has been considerable, a transfusion may even be necessary. Instead of a wanted pregnancy the woman will find herself having to contend with the loss of one of her two Fallopian tubes (and possibly an ovary as well), with pain, stitches and an unsightly scar (although thankfully this fades in time and does not pose any problem for future pregnancies). Vaginal bleeding is normal following the end of an ectopic pregnancy and the use of tampons should be avoided for a while because of the risk of infection, although it should be safe to use them by the time of the first period. Intercourse can normally resume once the woman feels physically and emotionally ready, although there may be pain at the site for some time afterwards and it is wise to avoid intercourse for at least four to six weeks following an ectopic pregnancy, to allow time for the body to heal.

The risk of a second ectopic pregnancy is unfortunately higher than in the average population. Some statistics quote 1 in every 30 conceptions, others suggest that it could be about 10 per cent (as against the general risk of 0.4 per cent). This last figure sounds depressing but it still means a 90 per cent chance of a normal pregnancy, and even those unlucky enough to experience ectopic pregnancy twice may still be able to have a successful subsequent pregnancy provided that they still have enough of a remaining tube for it to function or if they are able to bear a child via *in vitro* fertilization.

Because we have two Fallopian tubes, losing one means that the other becomes very precious and the fear that another conception may result in another ectopic pregnancy and the loss of the remaining tube is very real indeed. *In vitro* fertilization is still only available to a fortunate few and at present has only a limited success rate. Many women cannot bear the thought that risking another pregnancy might prove to be their last chance of bearing a child and it takes great courage to embark upon another pregnancy after experiencing one that was ectopic.

Both the physical and the emotional aftermath of ectopic pregnancy are considerable and should not be underestimated. In instances like this it is helpful when the media or programmes such as television and radio 'soap operas' draw attention to the issues involved. Shula Archer's experience of ectopic pregnancy in *The Archers* probably did more to advance public awareness, evoke sympathy and promote understanding than any amount of medical literature could have done. There is a danger, of course, that tragedies such as miscarriage and cot death can be exploited by soap operas simply as a cynical way of boosting the ratings, but when such events are handled accurately and sensitively they can be of genuine benefit to those affected by them in real life.

Hydatidiform mole

'Hydatid' means 'watery cyst' and in the very rare condition of hydatidiform mole the placenta grows very rapidly, producing a mass of cysts which resemble small grapes in appearance. According to one set of statistics, the risk is 1 in 1000 conceptions; according to another, the risk is 1 in 2000. The problem is thought to arise when an 'empty' ovum (i.e. lacking the essential genetic material) is fertilized by a normal sperm. Recent work by Dr Gudrun Moore, of Queen Charlotte's Hospital, suggests that two sperm fertilizing an empty egg may be responsible. As the rapid growth of the placenta leads to an increase in hormone levels, the woman concerned is likely to experience severe nausea and vomiting and may develop high blood pressure. Her uterus is likely to be 'large for dates' and she may experience vaginal bleeding, sometimes very dark and described as 'prune-coloured'.

If a molar pregnancy is suspected, an ultrasound scan will reveal its presence as a 'snowstorm' on the screen. Such pregnancies are usually diagnosed at about 16 weeks and must be terminated immediately under general anaesthetic, with great care taken to ensure that the uterus is completely emptied. If miscarriage has already taken place, then a D and C should still be performed, to ensure the same outcome. This is important because if any tissue from the mole remains in the uterus it may continue to grow and become cancerous – a condition known as choriocarcinoma. Thankfully this is usually completely curable provided it is caught in time. Because of the related risk, women who have had a hydatidiform mole are checked frequently in the months which follow. These checks are easily done, using blood and urine samples to ensure that hormone levels return to normal and remain stable (a raise in the level of the pregnancy hormone HCG would indicate that molar tissue was still growing in the womb whereas a consistent level would reassure that all was well).

At one time women experiencing hydatidiform mole were advised to wait two years before conceiving again but now, if the test results remain normal for six months, they may be allowed to try again sooner. They carry a 1 in 75 risk of another molar pregnancy (some say 1 in 50) and it does have a slight tendency to run in families, but even if it occurs again the chances of a subsequent straightforward pregnancy remain good.

Like ectopic pregnancy, hydatidiform mole carries with it specific shock and trauma: first, of learning that the anticipated baby never existed – that all the signs of pregnancy were a cruel delusion, and second, of learning of the risk of subsequent cancer. When Amanda discovered that tests on the tissue extracted during her D and C had confirmed the presence of a hydatidiform mole, understandably she wanted to know about the implications and so she went to a bookshop with a good medical section:

I discovered hydatidiform moles are benign but proliferative tumours, that they occur in 1 in 1000 pregnancies in the West and that they look like tiny clusters of grapes. I already knew that they were pre-cancerous in 10 per cent of cases. Now I learned that the resulting cancer in those cases was highly malignant and had to be pre-empted by chemotherapy or hysterectomy. Tumour . . . chemotherapy . . . hysterectomy . . . ME? . . . at 29? My alarm was further fuelled by the arrival of my first letter from Charing Cross Hospital. It was on paper headed with the logo of Cancer Research Campaign and it informed me that I was now a patient of their oncology department.

Once a fortnight, for weeks afterwards, Amanda had to attend her local hospital for a blood test and to send the serum and urine sample for analysis, until the welcome day arrived when she was informed that her hormone levels were back to normal – the mole had gone.

Suddenly a colossal burden had lifted, a burden whose weight I only really understood at that moment. I felt as if I had been given permission to live.

Knowing that the baby was never there in no way reduces the grief for that baby. As Amanda points out:

When you have a molar pregnancy you lose your identity as a mother-to-be, all the hopes that any expectant mother has and the opportunity usually available after miscarriage to try again within two or three months. And you have to wonder about cancer.

Thankfully hydatidiform mole is very rare, but that is of little comfort to those unlucky enough to find themselves having to cope with it and they will need help, support and good listeners in the months that follow.

Likely physical after-effects of a miscarriage

Even when physical recovery is rapid, this can seem like a mixed blessing because it means that all evidence of the pregnancy soon vanishes, leaving the mother feeling empty and cheated. The bleeding normally stops completely after two or three weeks, sometimes sooner. While it continues, sanitary towels should be used not tampons because of the increased risk of infection while the cervix remains open. It is, however, safe to shower as often as you wish or take a bath after 3–5 days. If the bleeding or discharge continues beyond three weeks, becomes heavier, contains clots or acquires an offensive smell, then you should contact your doctor as these are indications that fragments of tissue may still be present in the uterus. You should also contact your doctor if you develop a temperature or experience pelvic pain or feel unwell, as these signs could indicate the presence of an infection requiring prompt treatment with antibiotics. After the physical trauma of a miscarriage the body often recovers with surprising speed, but do allow for extra tiredness and grant your body a time of healing, resting whenever you feel the need to do so. The same holds true for those recovering from a D and C operation. All operations involve a degree of physical trauma and the body needs time to recover both from the effects of the operation and from the accompanying anaesthetic.

Most doctors advise waiting until the bleeding has stopped before resuming lovemaking, because of the possibility of increased risk of infection. The depression which commonly follows a miscarriage can cause a loss of libido and you may find that you do not wish to make love for a while, but on the other hand the sense of mutual loss can often bring a couple closer together and they may find themselves wanting to make love as a source of shared comforting. If you want to make love but not conceive for a while, then it is important to remember that you can ovulate at any time following a miscarriage and that therefore some form of contraception will be necessary. It would be wise to wait at least 6 weeks before having a coil (IUD) fitted, because the uterus will still be somewhat soft and there is an increased risk of perforation during insertion. Likewise, if you normally use a diaphragm then you would need to have the size checked as your own size may have altered because of the miscarriage. Condoms can be used straightaway, however, and the Pill can be started on the day after the miscarriage if you so wish, although of course there will be a lapse of 14 days before it becomes effective.

As far as periods are concerned, these usually begin again about a month after the miscarriage, but this can vary. (After my late miscarriage in May 1974 I continued to bleed until the July and then had to have a D and C operation. The doctor then advised us to allow three normal periods before trying for another baby, so we allowed the July, August and September periods to pass and then I was lucky enough to become pregnant straightaway in October. After my early miscarriage in June 1984, on the other hand, it took a full six months for my periods to truly re-establish and settle into their former pattern, enabling me to become pregnant again in early January 1985.)

After a late miscarriage, your body will need time to recover just as it would after a full-term labour and birth. Late miscarriages are usually followed up by an appointment at the hospital or with your GP, 4–6 weeks after the baby's delivery, to check your physical recovery, discuss the results of any post-mortem or tests and to answer any queries. The physical and emotional shock of the miscarriage can lower your body's resistance to infection and so it is worth making a conscious effort to build up your health through temporary vitamin and mineral supplements and through good, balanced meals even though you may not feel like eating at the time; alternatively, of course, you may find yourself in danger of 'comfort eating'. It is also worth remembering that temporary anaemia is a possibility following long and heavy blood loss, and this can cause sleeplessness and a 'tight' feeling in your throat, as well as making you feel very run-down and tired, so again a temporary iron supplement is worth considering. Floradix is a useful iron supplement. It is a very effective herbal iron preparation, recommended by midwives, which is easily absorbed and it can be obtained from most health food shops.

In later miscarriages, the baby is very real and recognizable and the mother is likely to be able to know whether she has lost a boy or a girl. Again, emotional reactions to late miscarriages can vary greatly and these will be discussed in the next chapter.

3
The Emotional Impact

How women view the nature of their loss does not necessarily correspond to the length of the pregnancy. Some women do not perceive the child they are carrying as a real baby until late in pregnancy or even until full-term delivery. Others view even the smallest embryo or fetus as a real baby. Women will only need to grieve if they perceive their miscarriage as a loss and some women don't, regarding an early miscarriage as little more than a late period. As they have not yet formed an emotional attachment and do not yet visualize the embryo or fetus as a baby or a potential person they are able to recover with few emotional ill-effects. Likewise, if they felt that something was definitely wrong with the pregnancy and that the miscarriage was the natural and right course of action for their bodies to take, then their feelings of loss are more likely to be minimized. The extent of the emotional impact will depend on your feelings towards your growing baby prior to the miscarriage, as well as on your reasons for becoming pregnant and your amount of emotional investment in the pregnancy, so don't feel guilty if you seem to be taking longer than others to recover. The greater the emotional investment in the pregnancy, the greater the emotional loss will feel when miscarriage occurs.

It is natural, in these days of good contraception and advanced medical care, to believe that the planning of our children is within our control and it can therefore come as a devastating shock to discover that this is not always the case. In some ways it is more difficult to adjust to miscarriage now because our expectations are so different. The main priority in previous centuries was often how to prevent too many births, and the expectation was that not all babies born alive would survive. Women were sometimes forced to take drastic measures to prevent conception or the continuation of yet another pregnancy. For women in financial poverty, dragged down physically and emotionally by relentless childbearing and facing the much greater risk of dying during childbirth (40 times more likely than the risk today), miscarriage may well have been viewed differently, in some ways a natural and sometimes welcome way of restricting the size of the family. In the 1990s, our expectations are very different. For those of us who only expect to experience two, possibly three, pregnancies throughout the whole of our reproductive life, those pregnancies become very precious indeed and our natural assumption is that each of the pregnancies will culminate in a healthy, live, full-term baby. The higher the expectation, the more shattering the experience when that expectation is not fulfilled.

My own experience

For the sake of clarity I made the decision to look separately at the physical and the emotional impact of miscarriage, but of course the two are intimately linked and how the physical experience is handled will affect the emotional consequences. Looking back now after 17 years to when our first little daughter came into this world too small and too young to survive, I still feel grief and anger that the pregnancy could suddenly have gone so wrong and that I was so ignorant and unprepared for the events which overtook me. I had been enjoying my first pregnancy so much, even admiring my ever-increasing outline in glass shop windows, revelling in the visible proof of my fertility and approaching motherhood. Oh, vanity. Our baby was due in August and when I took ill in the May with 'flu-like symptoms I did not worry unduly except that when I tottered out of bed afterwards my tummy seemed much, much bigger. I went to my antenatal clinic on the Monday afterwards for my appointment and was admitted immediately to a hospital ward 'for observation'. I spent from the Monday to the following Saturday with intermittent pains (in and out of labour but I did not know it at the time), while daily tape measurements confirmed that I was continuing to swell until it looked as if my tummy button must burst from the sheer pressure. I was told that for some reason my amniotic fluid was increasing out of control, hence the rapid increase in size. The doctor was reluctant to drain off the excess fluid as he felt that it might trigger full labour, so the hospital adopted a 'wait and see' policy and I spent the week alternately hoping for the best and fearing the worst.

The sooner we are told the truth, the sooner we can begin to adjust to it. Holding out false hopes simply increases the distress when those hopes are not realized. By now I was 27 weeks and desperately wanted our baby to survive, but it was 1974 and there was a lack of special care facilities at the time. I therefore respected the nurse who was truthful enough to warn me that survival was very unlikely at that stage and I found that I was able to place trust in her because of her honesty. By the Saturday I was in severe pain, but for the nurse who tried to delude me into believing that these labour pains were simply a kidney infection, I felt neither trust nor respect. Never having been in labour I did not know that backache labour could exist but I do know that enduring it made that Saturday the longest, most lonely and most painful of my life.

My husband and mother came to visit, felt powerless, gave what support they could and then left. Of the staff I saw very little indeed, being left to my own devices in a side-room to cope with my 'kidney infection'. By evening the pain was making everything seem unreal. I started to apologize to our little baby in my mind, saying how much I loved and wanted to keep him or her safely inside and promising to fight my own body for as long as I could. In my head she answered me, told me that she was a girl, told me her name (not one I would have chosen and one that I have never revealed to anyone because I find it so intensely private), told me that she understood why she was having to be born now and told me not to grieve for her because she didn't need this life. It was very clear and very comforting. At 10.45 p.m. my strength finally gave out. I can remember clearly saying to my baby: 'I'm sorry, I can't fight any more' and at that moment my waters gave, with a gushing that swamped the bed. Because my amniotic fluid had been multiplying totally out of control all week, there was fluid everywhere and when I lay back in bed to press the alarm bell my hair, my nightdress and the bed became completely soaked. When the night nurse arrived she panicked at the sight which confronted her. She told me to sit on the edge of the bed, but the resulting dip made all the fluid spill onto the floor, mingling with the water from my vase of flowers which she had knocked over in her confusion. She then made me sit in a chair and began to strip the bed! Because my labour had been denied, nothing was prepared, least of all myself. She could not find my notes, she could not find the doctor on duty, I was unbathed, unshaven and my bowels were decidedly full. By then I knew that the birth was imminent because I could feel the baby's head, but having transferred me into a wheelchair, she then abandoned me while she went for help, leaving me alone in a corridor convinced that my baby was going to be born into the chair or onto the cold hospital floor. My body was insisting on pushing despite all my attempts to stop it and I was very, very frightened. When the nurse returned there followed a nightmare journey through hospital corridors to the delivery room. I remember the appalled look on the face of an anxious young father-to-be as we emerged round a corner and I was rushed past him, drenched with fluid and shivering with shock and fear. God knows what the poor man must have thought of such a vision hurtling past him. Nor did the situation improve once we were in the delivery room because when two doctors arrived to deliver my baby, one proved to be an Egyptian man and the other an Indian lady, both apparently incapable of understanding each other. I realized that I could understand most of what the Egyptian doctor was saying and at one point found myself lying on the delivery bed, acting as interpreter and thinking: 'This can't be real, it can't be happening'. When I saw the Indian doctor with scalpel poised and realized that she was asking whether to conduct an episiotomy, I gave one final and very determined push and brought our little daughter into the world.

I never really saw her. I had an agonizing glimpse of our daughter as they lifted her up and wrapped her in a dark green towel and then she was whisked away for resuscitation. By then a sister had arrived. When she came back to me from the resuscitation room her face was grave. She explained that my baby's heart had still been beating after delivery but that she had never breathed independently and had not survived. Interestingly, at no time did anyone refer to her as a spontaneous abortion, although 'abortion' is what was entered later in my hospital notes. The nursing sister began talking about the definitions of stillbirth and live birth, explaining that if we wanted to class her as a live birth we would have to undergo the trauma of a post-mortem and inquest and all the expense of a funeral and was that what I really wanted? By then I had gone into surgical shock, teeth chattering uncontrollably and in no state to make any rational decisions. As far as I was concerned, my baby was dead and I didn't want to fight to live, I just wanted to give up and die too so that at least I could be with her. I heard someone say that I was toxic, whatever that meant, and someone else sent out an urgent message for blankets, to try and stop me from shivering so much. Incredibly they couldn't find any! As it had been a warm week in May I suppose the staff had felt that there would be no call for blankets, but the delay in finding any merely compounded the severity of the surgical shock, and for days afterwards my teeth and jaws ached from the effects of the severe and uncontrollable shivering.

After writing this account for the book, I hunted for and found what I had written at the time. I had done so as a way of trying to come to terms with what had happened. I had not looked at it in 17 years. My memory was uncomfortably perfect. It still seems like a nightmare, one that continues to make me angry when I allow myself to think about it because so much of it could have been avoided. Either the day staff genuinely did not realize that I was in classic backache labour or for misguided reasons they chose to ignore it. Recognizing and acknowledging it would have done much to prepare me emotionally for what lay ahead and would have enabled the staff to prepare me physically for giving birth. At that time the routine procedure was to wash and shave mothers-to-be and give an enema. As it was, I had to suffer the grumbles of the doctor who had to wait while I was shaved on the delivery table in the midst of my contractions, followed by the humiliation of being unable to prevent my bowels from evacuating during the birth. The nurse who had to deal with what by night-time had become a medical emergency was far too young and inexperienced to cope and should never have been left in charge without support. Her panic and fear transferred all too easily to me during what was already a very new and frightening experience. Having two doctors incapable of understanding each other did little to provide re-assurance, either. I have to hope that hospital treatment of mothers who are miscarrying has improved in the last 17 years.

I've related what happened to me, partly because it has helped me to do so after all this time and partly because I hope that it may be of help to others as well, encouraging women to talk about their experiences and press for improvements. A caring attitude does not cost money and what I had needed and failed to receive was support from staff who could acknowledge my labour, give me accurate and honest information as to what to expect and help me through the experience. Mothers who lose their babies are well aware that it is a distressing situation for staff to handle, but they do need support and towards nurses who *are* able to offer help and advice they feel lasting respect and gratitude.

Grieving

Those of us who perceive our miscarriage as a bereavement will grieve, whether or not we are aware of it at the time. There are no right or wrong reactions to bereavement, only natural ones. At times we will cope, at other times we won't, but the process of grieving will continue until we have worked our way through it and I know from experience that there are no short-cuts. However 'brave' we may try to be and however much we may try to suppress our feelings, sooner or later they will surface and we will have to face and deal with them in order to heal and move on from our experience. I have learnt this truth the hard way. Following the loss of our first daughter, my next pregnancy was successful and our lovely daughter Rebecca was born in 1975. All went well and in 1979 I was overjoyed to discover that I was expecting twins. Elizabeth and Mary were born seven weeks prematurely in June 1979. It was a very anxious time, but they survived and made good progress and after five weeks in intensive care they were able to come home, to a very special, brief but precious time. On the morning of 6th September, when she was 3 months old, I found Elizabeth dead in her pram. No warning, nothing – a cot death. Grieving for her culminated in the writing of my first book, *Coping with Cot Death*, but I also know that the truths I learnt from her death apply to miscarriage as well and that grieving after miscarriage is just as natural and necessary, so I make no apology for planning to include one or two quotes from *Coping with Cot Death* which have equal relevance here.

We are all individuals and therefore our reactions are unique to ourselves, but the hard work of grieving does seem to have certain stages and it can help to be forewarned of likely reactions with which you may find yourself having to cope. The most recognized are: numbing, followed by disbelief, followed by disorganization and finally by reorganization, which may take months or even years to achieve. As these are such important aspects following a miscarriage, I think the best way to approach them will be to talk about the initial two 'stages' in this chapter and the later two 'stages' in the next chapter: 'Coping From Within'. Obviously there are no set rules where grieving is concerned, just likely reactions and responses. One mistake I made was to assume that grief, because it has a definite beginning, must also have a definite end, that there would come a time when I could say: 'There, we're through it and it's over'. I know now that grief has no end. We can learn to reorganize and to adjust our lives but it seems likely that the grief, though it alters as we alter, will always remain part of us. As someone has pointed out, our experience of miscarriage is not an obstacle to be 'got over', it is an integral part of ourselves and how should we 'get over' being ourselves?

Numbing and shock

Most of us who find ourselves suddenly experiencing a miscarriage will be far too busy coping with the actual physical trauma to allow ourselves to take on board any of the emotional implications until afterwards. As far as the first stage of numbing is concerned, the shock is almost a help because it acts as an anaesthetic. It is when the initial shock wears off that the real, physical pain of heartache begins. You may find yourself being offered tranquillizers. Whilst it may be tempting to accept, these only postpone the pain, they don't remove it. If you feel that prolonging the period of numbness may help, then by all means accept the use of tranquillizers, but you will have to accept, too, that sooner or later the reality of your baby's death has to be faced and grieving allowed to begin. The use of alcohol may also deaden the pain for a while but, again, this is only a temporary effect and not a long-term solution. As someone once neatly put it: 'I drank to drown my sorrows, but they soon all learnt how to swim'.

Responses to the initial shock and bereavement are likely to vary. Some of us may feel a strong need for company, the physical comfort and reassurance of others around us, but some of us may need to shut ourselves away for a while. When our first daughter died I wanted, like an animal, to crawl away somewhere very private to lick my emotional wounds, but in hospital this was not possible (see p. 88 for further details concerning this problem which many bereaved mothers encounter). Even after my return home a week later, I still wanted to hide, paradoxically wanting support from my husband Pat but also wanting privacy, so that I lay in bed, not wanting him to disturb me yet resenting the fact that he was downstairs watching television. Irrational emotions are certainly one of the consequences of miscarriage!

When miscarriage does take place, some women experience a brief period almost of relief and elation that the miscarriage is finally over and that they've survived, but this is often then followed by a period of very real depression as the full implications of the loss become apparent. The loss of our baby includes the loss of all the associated events which would have accompanied and followed the birth and we have to grieve for them, too. Because the loss is so great, it can rekindle previous losses and leave us trying to cope with reawakened, unresolved griefs as well.

A feeling of emptiness is very common after a miscarriage, both in a literal physical way because the baby is no longer inside us, but also in an emotional way. For some, the emptiness can be long-lasting. It is as if we set aside a whole part of ourselves ready to receive all the experiences and memories we are looking forward to sharing with our son or daughter right through from babyhood and childhood to adolescence and adulthood and when that baby is born too soon and does not survive, that part of us may remain an emptiness which can never be truly filled again.

Disbelief

For a while you may well find that you simply can't accept what has happened. How can the world carry on so normally, buses moving, people shopping, when your own particular world has been so completely shattered? The urge to turn back the clock to when everything was all right can be very strong indeed and can leave you feeling angry and powerless when it can't be done. Those of us who experience missed abortion or blighted ovum have an extra stark reality to bear – that the baby we thought was growing inside us and with whom we felt closeness and communication has been dead for some time or indeed was never even there. This harsh realization does not in any way invalidate our feelings. If our baby was real to us then our loss and our need to mourn will also be real, so we must allow ourselves to do so.

Part of the difficulty in coping with disbelief is that our natural mothering instincts do not die with the death of our baby. Many of us experience an intense physical aching to hold the baby who is no longer there – especially if we find ourselves producing milk – together with a desire to protect our baby from harm. I can remember that in the first few weeks after our daughter was miscarried, I continued to move very carefully in my sleep, as if she was still inside me, only to waken to the bitter realization of my new and unwelcome flatness. A friend of mine, whose toddler died in a very late cot death, told me that at his burial she wanted more than anything else to lay a blanket on his grave to keep him warm. This desire to protect is very natural and it is one of the reasons why the cliché of miscarriage being 'nature's way of removing damaged or abnormal fetuses' is of little comfort. Hearing our potential babies being condemned as imperfect fetuses and not fit to live can arouse very strong maternal instincts indeed.

The same maternal instinct can make it very difficult for us to leave the hospital afterwards, as if we are somehow betraying and abandoning our baby. We may find ourselves wanting to search for our baby even though we know that he or she is dead and if we deny this urge it is likely to reappear in our dreams or nightmares, which tend to be common following miscarriage.

Even early miscarriage leaves us with unanswerable questions. As Carol expressed it:

> If a heartbeat can be found as early as 6 or 7 weeks, then the fetus has a heart, so does it also have a soul? Did it go to Heaven? Will I meet it when I die? I know these questions can't be answered, but I ask myself the same questions over and over again.

Mothers who miscarry one baby during a twin or multiple pregnancy are left with the baffling question: 'Why? Why did one of my babies die and will my surviving baby (or babies) be safe and well?' Those of you who find yourselves in such a situation may feel torn between the desire to focus on your surviving baby (or babies) and the need to mourn your baby who has been lost. For you, the chapters which follow will be just as necessary and relevant as for those who experience miscarriage during a single pregnancy, for you, too, will find yourselves experiencing the natural grief reactions which, as mentioned, tend to begin with numbing and disbelief.

One of the ways in which we try to cope with our feelings of disbelief is by going over and over what has happened, the way that we might rub our tongue over and over a tooth that is aching. Such repetition may be hard for partners, relatives and friends to endure, but it is a very necessary part of trying to accept the reality of what has happened. So, too, are tears and some of us may wonder if the crying will ever stop, but it is an essential part of grieving, so never try to suppress it for the sake of others; this is one occasion when your own needs must come first.

4

Coping From Within

Much of the hard work of grieving happens inside us, in our hearts and minds and souls, and that's why I am devoting a separate chapter to this process of 'coping from within'.

Disorganization

This is the longest part of grieving and you may find yourself having to cope with a frightening array of very powerful emotions, some of them previously totally alien to you. In part, of course, such emotions can be the result of all the hormonal disruption caused by the miscarriage. It is difficult enough having to cope with a form of postnatal depression when there is the positive reward of a baby to love; having the depression without the baby is very hard indeed.

Depression
Amanda, who lost her twin daughters at 23 weeks, wrote:

> No warning given by hospital or GP that I was likely to feel profoundly depressed for a good year after. No information given about support groups. The result was that we didn't realize how normal my reaction was. I wasted a huge amount of nervous energy trying to 'get over it' when I would have done better to accept my feelings and let them take their course.

Depression is a natural response to bereavement, sometimes accompanied by a temporary feeling of utter despair where nothing seems to matter any more. Some of us may not even realize that we are trying to cope with depression, and as a result may feel that we are having some sort of breakdown or even going mad – a very frightening prospect. If we and those around us fail to recognize the signs of depression, it can worsen and become severe. It is helpful to know that some of the classic signs of depression are perpetual weakness and tiredness (often accompanied by an inability to sleep), weepiness, erratic and sometimes violent mood changes, inability to concentrate, loss of interest in everything and everyone around you and a feeling that a heavy black weight is literally pressing down upon you and encompassing you, leaving you feeling trapped within and unable to escape. Instead of being full of colour, the world becomes grey and meaningless. If you do find yourself experiencing these or other symptoms, do be brave enough to talk about what you are feeling and experiencing and to consult your doctor if you feel that severe depression may be threatening to engulf you.

During this phase, everything seems not merely trivial and pointless but also an incredible physical effort and you may find yourself functioning purely on auto-pilot and feeling totally over-powered by a relentless tiredness. Since memory and concentration are also likely to be severely affected, this can be very difficult when you are trying to look after your family and home, especially if you are also working. If, on the other hand, you had just stopped work in anticipation of the birth or you decide to wait before returning to work afterwards, then you can find yourself feeling completely disorientated by being in an empty, silent house where former occupations such as vacuuming and cleaning suddenly seem totally fatuous and futile. (For more about the problems which may be encountered when deciding whether to stay at home or return to work, see pp. 79–81.)

Anger

It is said that depression is anger turned inwards upon itself. In that case, I know that I must have been very angry at times! It showed itself outwardly in brief flashes of fury over trivial incidents, fury which tended to erupt and then subside as quickly as it came. To reduce the risk of depression, perhaps it is better to allow our anger to have outward expression and to work through it rather than try to deny or suppress it. Many women do this unconsciously by directing their natural feelings of anger outwards, towards their doctor, the hospital staff, pregnant women, Fate or God. (It is even natural to feel angry with our baby for seeming to reject us by being born too soon and leaving us, but in that case we are likely to feel guilty at such anger and to deny it both to ourselves and to others.)

Whilst we may feel ashamed and guilty about our anger, it can be a positive emotion, helping us to overcome feelings of being a victim and of being powerless. Sometimes anger against the doctor or hospital staff may be justified – when care has been inappropriate or inadequate – and such anger can be the motivating force which leads to future improvements in care.

Many people find that they have feelings of anger towards God, and some of us may see our miscarriage as a rejection by God or as a punishment for some sin which knowingly or unknowingly we may have committed in the past. Having thought about this in *Coping with Cot Death*, I realize now that it is just as relevant where miscarriage is concerned. When we miscarry and our baby dies, we can feel sheer helpless rage that we are unable to save our baby and since for believers God is the giver of life, then this rage may direct itself against God as being the taker of life as well. God can handle our anger, he knows all about it. Far from condemning us, he will help us work through it if we are totally honest with him and allow him to do so. To make room for healing and love to come in, we have to let the hurt and anger out, so don't try to deny it or bottle it up inside, yell it out. Go somewhere private and scream and shout, punch cushions, tear up cardboard boxes, smash plates, anything that will exorcize the anger which, if left inside you, may fester and poison for years to come. If expressing yourself in such a way is not natural or easy for you, try flinging it all onto canvas in paintings or set it all down on paper in drawings or in writing. When Judy Gordon Morrow finally acknowledged her anger at losing her baby and wrote down all her feelings, she discovered that her handwriting even *looked* angry. Afterwards she felt drained but more at peace. Her sister astutely observed later that:

> Judy didn't realize that when she wrote out her anger and threw her questions at God, she stood in a very biblical tradition. In the Bible – particularly in the Psalms, the prophets, and in Job – we see people who questioned God, complained, challenged, and protested. And we don't sense that they were far from God, but rather just the opposite. They were close enough to trust him with all of their feelings, not just the ones that they deemed acceptable.
>
> And their angry, questioning, complaining words became their prayers, the means by which they connected with God. And instead of distancing them from God, the words brought them closer. In wrestling with God, they ended up experiencing his embrace. (*Good Mourning*, Word UK, 1989)

As I feel that it might be helpful, I will quote below what I wrote in *Coping with Cot Death*. I'm only amazed that it has taken the writing of this book to make me recognize something so obvious, that what applied to Elizabeth was true of our first baby as well and I could not see it until now:

'The Lord giveth and the Lord taketh away, blessed be the name of the Lord.' I couldn't accept it. *Why? Why* had he given, only to take away? It was five years later that a Christian friend, Chris, advised me to give both Elizabeth and my grief to God and I realized a truth – grief is not only supremely self-centred, it is also possessive. I still wanted Elizabeth and I still wanted my grief; they were mine. And then thankfully, for me, the problem resolved itself. It was not that God had taken Elizabeth, simply that he had been there to receive her when she went. A phrase from schooldays came back to me, from a poem by Wilfred Owen about soldiers going 'over the top' into battle in the First World War: 'Some say God caught them even before they fell'. I had never doubted Elizabeth's place in heaven. Now at last I could see that she hadn't been taken, she had been received.

This insight into God as being supportive and loving and receiving instead of as punishing and snatching away has been of profound help to me concerning Elizabeth's death. But up until now, I realize that I have never accepted our first baby's going, nor have I been willing to give her to God and that I've resented him for having her because even though she may not have needed this life, *I* needed her. Maybe I've even been feeling rejected by her at a very deep level indeed that she didn't need me and didn't stay. If she had stayed, we wouldn't now have Rebecca, who has brought us so much happiness and who this week is at home in Sussex, looking after Mary and Christopher after school each day while Pat is at work, so that I can be here in the privacy and peace of this Welsh cottage, writing about miscarriage and about her older sister whom none of us ever had the chance to know. Strange indeed.

Miscarriage brings us face to face with very basic and crucial issues surrounding life and death, and sadly, their experience of miscarriage can lead some couples to reject their former faith, but equally it can also lead some to an increase in faith because death is such a very primal experience which puts us in touch both with ourselves and with what is eternal.

Believing in God does not reduce the grieving, however, and can lead some to feel guilty that their faith has not shielded them from mourning. Guilt again. How often the word emerges when talking about miscarriage!

Why me?

Our anger is usually accompanied by feelings of bitter disappointment, of hopes crushed and a sense of 'Why me?' because miscarriage is truly a miscarriage of justice. We may also find ourselves having to cope with a whole host of unexpected and unpleasant emotions such as a feeling of definite rivalry with women who are pregnant. Our feelings towards such women can encompass deep envy and jealousy which can border on violence, hate and rage that they are being allowed what we have been denied. Carol wrote:

> I was very shocked by the depth of my feelings. I don't show my emotions easily, but I had no control over the grief, anger, hurt and hate that I felt. The hatred was directed at pregnant women, I'm afraid.

Similarly Debbie wrote:

> I couldn't bear to go out and see pregnant women and babies.

and Carol added in her letter:

> I'm beginning to wonder if there'll ever be a time when babies, pregnant women and my period don't upset me.

All these emotions, of course, simply compound our sense of guilt and they can be very difficult to handle, especially if we never even knew that we were capable of them and feel shocked at their depth and intensity. The world can suddenly seem to be full of pregnant women – strangers in the street or women known to us who may add insult to injury by grumbling about their pregnancies. The deep yearning to have another baby which many of us feel can be very strong and can even make some of us fear that we may steal any baby we see left unattended.

If a close friend or relative is expecting a baby at about the time that yours would have been due then this can be especially hard to bear, not least because of the long-term implications involved in watching the progress of the surviving child, comparing and thinking about what might have been. If you already have older children then escape is impossible because your daily routine is going to involve mother-and-toddler group, playgroup, nursery or school, with the inevitable sight of babies, small children and groups of waiting mothers, some of whom are bound to be mothers-in-waiting.

Guilt and self-blame

Thankfully there are indications that the temptation to blame our own actions for our miscarriage has lessened in the light of increased medical knowledge, and there are signs that we are now willing to be more open-minded about the possible causes of miscarriage and less ready to blame ourselves or our immediate circumstances. For some of us, however, guilt will always be a problem. It is a very common response following termination for abnormality. Anyone undergoing this is still losing a wanted baby. Feeling that she has made the right decision in no way diminishes her grief afterwards. Similarly, anyone who has had a previous induced abortion for whatever reason may find that subsequent miscarriage stirs up memories and unresolved feelings of guilt. Alternatively, of course, some may find themselves experiencing feelings which confirm that the earlier abortion was the right decision at the time. When guilt is aroused, however, some women may even feel that their previous history of abortion has caused the miscarriage despite the fact that, according to one study, there is less than a 4 per cent risk of this being the case. Keeping this in mind can help when coping with such feelings of guilt. Sometimes our ingenuity in finding metaphorical sticks with which to beat ourselves after a miscarriage knows no bounds. Did we cause it by continuing to work or alternatively by giving up work, thereby altering our routine? Did we cause it by moving house, or alternatively by staying in the house which may now seem jinxed? Did we cause the miscarriage because we decorated, or stretched up to hang curtains, or lifted heavy weights? If we feel guilty because we did something out of necessity, we are likely to feel even more guilty if we were doing something for enjoyment – 'I should never have gone on holiday/made love/gone for that game of tennis/jog/climb/ride/swim'. The fact that there is absolutely no evidence to suggest that any of these activities has any link with subsequent miscarriage does little to allay our sense of guilt. We need to find a cause, something to blame, if only to try and prevent it from happening again, and in the absence of any other apparent cause the tendency is to blame ourselves. We may even worry in case we have somehow unconsciously rejected our baby in the womb during the very mixed emotions of pregnancy, or failed to love our baby sufficiently for him or her to survive. This can be especially true if the pregnancy was unplanned, and it merely compounds the sense of guilt which follows the miscarriage, no matter how unjustified that may be. There is no easy way to handle a feeling of guilt except to recognize it for what it is, and to try and hold on to the realization that it is neither warranted nor necessary.

Loss of self-esteem and self-confidence

Miscarriage for some of us can be our first major experience of 'failure' and it happens in such a crucial area of our lives – potential motherhood. When we miscarry our first baby no sooner do we discover the importance of the status of pregnancy and motherhood to society and (perhaps as a complete surprise) to ourselves than we lose it. No one should underestimate the power which miscarriage has to alter and sometimes severely damage our own image of and belief in ourselves. Some of us will already have a child or children when we experience miscarriage and at least we will have the reassurance of knowing that we are able to have children and that, having had successful pregnancies before, we can hope to have another successful pregnancy in the future. Parents who lose their first baby have no such reassurance and as a result may find their confidence severely undermined. Even though the next pregnancy may well be successful, any subsequent baby will not be their first baby and therefore that is a very special loss. No subsequent pregnancy can ever recapture the excitement and magic of the first and any future pregnancy is likely to be fearfully endured rather than confidently enjoyed. This is, of course, also true of mothers who already have children. Once a pregnancy fails, being pregnant can never be the same experience again.

A mother who already has children may be helped by the fact that they will tend to keep her busy and give her a sense of purpose following her miscarriage, but she may also find that their needs can be an added stress and that trying to comfort and reassure them will sap her own precarious reserves of physical and emotional energy. It can be very difficult trying to explain your miscarriage to others in your family when you are finding it impossible to understand it yourself. From anticipating motherhood and a baby, we are suddenly left with neither, only an overwhelming sense of failure

51

and of betrayal by our own bodies – plus a feeling of having failed everyone else around us: our partner, our parents for being deprived of a potential grandchild, our existing children for being deprived of a younger brother or sister. The arranged spacing between our children, which may have seemed so right at the time, is suddenly gone and can never be regained. No matter what the future holds, it will not be the one we planned.

All at once nothing can be taken for granted any more – not even our own fertility; life ceases to hold guarantees. We begin to realize that if pregnancy can go wrong, maybe other aspects of our life may go wrong as well and this can badly threaten our sense of security. Some of us who had thought ourselves strong and capable suddenly discover that we are very vulnerable indeed, prone to violent mood swings, which might previously have been totally out of character, and struggling to cope with emotions well beyond our control. It can be a very chastening experience and it can alter the way we see both ourselves and others. As we begin to pick up the pieces and adjust, one of the realities which we have to accept is that we can never be the same person again. Part of that person died with the baby and the subsequent person we become has to let go not only of the baby but of the person we used to be as well.

Loss of illusions and innocence about pregnancy

We are so surrounded by images of joyous pregnancy and fulfilling motherhood in magazines and on television that we may not even be aware of how much they influence our expectations until something goes wrong. Where are the magazine articles or antenatal clinic literature that could tell us just how often miscarriage happens and forewarn us of the possibility? Miscarriage is a negative aspect of pregnancy and therefore it is regarded as unacceptable, something which must be kept hidden, as if denying it could somehow mean that it does not exist. We know to our cost that it does, and pretending otherwise acts as a grave disservice to all those thousands of women each year who find themselves coping with both the experience and its aftermath. In trying to protect expectant mothers from anxiety by not alerting them to the high incidence of miscarriage, those who do miscarry are left totally unprotected and unprepared. Surely, forewarned is forearmed! We all experience major life changes from time to time. The ones to which it is most difficult for us to adjust are the ones that come as a total shock, catching us completely unaware and unprepared. Is there perhaps something patronizing in the implication that as expectant mothers we are incapable of coping with information about miscarriage? Accurate facts would enable us to make informed decisions regarding our lifestyles during pregnancy, which if nothing else might reduce the tendency to blame ourselves when miscarriage occurs, for something we did or did not do. 'If only' can be a very destructive game to play.

Of course no one wants to detract from the thrill of being pregnant nor to make young mothers-to-be anxious, but a realistic approach to pregnancy and miscarriage would at least make us aware that not all pregnancies will be successful. It is the absence of such awareness that makes miscarriage so hard to bear when our naive sense of innocence is lost and our illusions shattered. No wonder we feel such failures, isolated exceptions to the golden rule of motherhood and automatically barred from the desirable and exclusive club which accompanies it.

I didn't only feel a failure at becoming a mother, I even felt a failure where labour was concerned. Our baby was born just before my mothercraft classes had been due to begin. I was totally ignorant about labour and no one forewarned me that labour at 27 weeks could be extremely painful because of the body's unreadiness to give birth. I can remember thinking that since I had found it so very painful with such a small baby, how on earth would I ever cope with a full-term, full-size baby? Others managed it, what was wrong with me? Down went my self-esteem, up went my feelings of failure and inadequacy.

When such feelings of failure and inadequacy threaten, it can help to list achievements, however small – actions you accomplish without even thinking about them: cooking meals on time, remembering to wash and iron requested items of clothing, collecting or dropping off children to the right place at the right time with the right accessories (PE kit/recorder/violin for school or card and present for the birthday party to which they've been invited). We may seem like failures to ourselves at times, but those around us often appreciate qualities in us of which we are not even aware, and it can help to realize that our family and friends do love and value us, even if they don't always say so!

'An outward and visible sign of an inward and spiritual grace'. A healthy full-term baby is an outward and visible sign of our success as a couple, proof that our relationship has succeeded physically and confirmation of the 'inward and spiritual grace' of human love.

It's as if we say to the world: 'Look, we love each other and here's the proof of our love, a new person created by our love'. Any imperfection or failure to carry the pregnancy to term may seem to some to imply that somehow such a love is flawed in some way, and this can be hard to bear.

Recurrent miscarriage

Trying to cope with the emotional impact of recurrent miscarriages poses very special problems and women who suffer from a succession of miscarriages can feel battered in every sense of the word. When our first daughter miscarried, I felt that perhaps I had atoned for some unknown failure or sin. Although I was fearful throughout my subsequent pregnancy, part of me clung to the hope that the pain and grief of the first had wiped clean an unknown slate and that I was entitled to my next baby and the happiness that she would bring. While part of me feared losing her before birth, part of me reassured myself that neither God nor Nature could be so cruel, and Rebecca's safe arrival after a full-term pregnancy seemed to affirm such a belief. When, four years later, our twin daughter Elizabeth died at the age of three months, I was totally devastated. How could such pain happen again? I had never expected my life to be entirely free from suffering, but surely losing one daughter was enough? I can certainly identify with those who cry: 'Why me?' because I did so, too. I can also identify with those who experience recurrent miscarriage, because when our surviving twin daughter Mary started school and we decided to risk having another baby, the joy of immediate conception was crushed at 8 weeks by the early miscarriage which I mentioned in the last chapter. After the death of our first baby and after Elizabeth's death I was grief-stricken and even now, I cannot pretend to have come to terms with losing our two daughters, only that I have learnt to live with their loss, which will always be part of me. After the early miscarriage I wasn't grief-stricken, I was angry – angry with myself, for carrying all those sacks of jumble for a cot-death jumble sale, thereby jeopardizing the tiny life within me (for I was convinced that the heavy lifting had been the cause of the miscarriage); angry with the irony that trying to raise funds to save other people's babies had cost me my own; angry that others seemed to be able to have trouble-free pregnancies and babies who survived while we had been hit yet again. Having fought through a very real depression following Elizabeth's death and having believed myself to be safely on the other side, back I slid, my fragile self-confidence shattered again and depression threatening to engulf me. Thankfully it didn't, but that was a miserable six months until my periods stabilized and I became pregnant with Christopher. Even then, he tried to arrive 10 weeks prematurely, I had to spend time in hospital and it was only as a result of excellent medical care that he was persuaded to stay in the right place until his allotted 40 weeks.

Because of my own anger I can understand the natural anger of women who miscarry more than once. I can also understand their feeling of being jinxed or their tendency to become fatalistic, convinced that another miscarriage is going to happen. I can even identify with the urge to deliberately distance themselves from any subsequent pregnancy, pretending it isn't happening as a protection against the risk of more pain and disappointment. I wish I could find something positive to say to anyone experiencing recurrent miscarriage, but the response I find myself wanting to give holds little consolation, for it is: 'I'm sorry, and you're right, it *isn't* fair'.

Miscarriage following infertility

Life is also very unfair when conception takes a long time to achieve and the resulting baby is then miscarried. Couples can feel almost destroyed by such an outcome and understandably dread the thought that it could take just as long to conceive the next time, with no guarantee of a happy outcome. It is a wretched situation in which to be, relieved only by the realization that the baby who miscarried is proof that you are indeed fertile and that you can conceive. Hold on to that, and take comfort from the reassurance that after one miscarriage, you have a 75 per cent chance of having a normal subsequent pregnancy, which shows that the odds are in your favour.

Miscarriage in later life

Miscarriage in later life can also be especially hard to bear. Women who miscarry in their forties are only too aware that it may have been their last chance to have a baby. Sometimes the pregnancy was an unplanned one. Having just adapted to the idea of having a baby in later life, it can be extremely difficult to then adjust to the realization that this may never now be the case. Miscarriage when nearing the menopause reinforces the harsh reality of getting older and the loss involved can seem very final indeed.

Reorganization

The more I come into contact with women who have coped with both birth and death, the more impressed I become. Women possess incredible inner resources and strengths but often they are unaware of them until faced with a crisis or tragedy. Mary, who suffered one miscarriage at 8 weeks, a second at 12 weeks and a missed abortion at 18 weeks, expressed it succinctly when she said:

> Women are strong. Men can carry physical weights, but it's the women who are best able to carry the emotional weights.

Allowing the grieving

Before we can begin to reorganize and recover, some of us need to be given permission to grieve, either by someone like our doctor, our partner, a relative or friend or even by ourselves. It is as if, because miscarriage is seen as a trivial event in medical terms, we feel that we are not entitled to grieve, even though, to us, the miscarriage is far from trivial. I know now that I have spent the last 17 years denying many of my feelings about the loss of our first daughter, as if I was not entitled to such feelings because it was 'only a miscarriage' and because I had experienced death before birth, not death after birth. As someone has quite rightly described it, that is 'the ultimate paradox'. Death before birth goes totally against the natural order of events and consequently it is not just others who want to shy away from such a concept; sometimes, perhaps, we ourselves do, too.

In many ways, a miscarriage isn't so much an end, it's more of a beginning, the beginning of a long process of mourning and adapting and learning about ourselves. As I stressed earlier, there are no short-cuts to grief, but there are milestones and you should award yourself a mental 'tick' each time you face and overcome a painful situation. Congratulating someone on her pregnancy, handling someone else's baby for the first time, attending a family christening, coping with the date when your baby should have been born, coping with the first Christmas when you know that your baby should be with you to enjoy it all but isn't and never will be . . . occasions such as these are very painful and difficult, but even the ones we dread the most can be faced and overcome, they do pass and each time it gets just a little easier. Sooner or later you'll find that you're able to laugh at a television programme without feeling somehow guilty about enjoying yourself. The single most crucial piece of advice which I would give to couples who have experienced a miscarriage and perceive it as a bereavement is this: *Allow yourselves to grieve.* Some of us may try to suppress our grief, others may try to postpone it, but eventually it has to be acknowledged and worked through. Don't try to deny it to yourself or to others. Not only may outsiders misinterpret and assume that you are perfectly all right and not in need of any help, but you deny yourself valuable opportunities to let out your feelings and grief won't be denied, it will simply resurface later in life in other and perhaps more damaging ways.

If, like me, you find it difficult to express your needs to others or feel that you have to spare them from your pain (thereby answering their needs but not your own), then it is worth considering the idea of expressing your feelings in some other way, through drawing, painting or writing. Keeping a journal can be a very helpful outlet for your feelings and will provide an accurate record for you to look back upon in later years, should you feel the wish to do so.

During the stage of reorganization it can help if you are able to provide yourself with some sort of structure and routine when everything seems to have fallen apart, but it is important to avoid the danger of deliberately becoming so busy that you leave yourself no time to grieve, for this merely postpones the grieving, it doesn't remove it. Grieving takes time. Be kind to yourself, be patient with yourself and realistic in your expectations and you will make progress without even necessarily realizing that you are doing so.

Creating memories

As part of the process of reorganization, it is very helpful if you can create memories for yourself. Naming the baby can help and even if it was an early miscarriage and you do not know what sex your baby would have been, you can still choose a name applicable to either sex (such as Francis/es, Leslie/ey, Robin/yn, or an abbreviation such as Jo, Pat or Chris) if doing so helps you to give your baby an identity and focus your feelings.

One of the most difficult problems of miscarriage is that often there is no tangible baby to mourn, no focus for our feelings and, where the sex of the lost baby is unknown, no identity for us to recognize and acknowledge. Although it may sound morbid, evidence suggests that seeing the dead fetus or baby can help us to accept the reality of what has happened and provide us with just such a focus for our emotions. It can also remove fears that the fetus or baby may have looked deformed in some way when we see that our baby, however tiny, was perfect. Many couples opt not to see their dead baby and their wishes should always be respected. Of those who do see, either by choice or because they had no choice at the time, few seem to regret the experience and most say how helpful they found it because it enabled them to say hello and goodbye to their baby. (See p. 92 for more on this.)

Just as it can be hard to mourn a baby who was unseen and intangible, so also it can be hard when you have felt your baby moving inside you or seen your baby on a screen during a scan. These experiences give the baby reality but it is a reality which reinforces the loss when miscarriage takes place.

Some couples like to create their own memorials at home by planting a rose bush or erecting a special plaque. Others may like to create mementoes by having a special box or scrapbook containing all the reminders of pregnancy – photos of when you were pregnant, photos of the baby taken during scans or taken after birth following a late miscarriage, congratulations cards, appointment cards, maybe even the identity bracelet you wore during your hospital stay. Some may find this a morbid response but as stressed before, there are no right or wrong responses to bereavement, only natural ones and others may find the creation of mementoes and memories very comforting and helpful.

Allowing mourning rituals

As mentioned in Chapter 2, you are entitled to hold your own informal cremation or burial in your own garden at home, but it is worth bearing in mind that you might move house in the future. Alternatively, having some form of official funeral can help you as a couple to acknowledge your loss and say goodbye to your baby and this can sometimes be arranged on either a religious or a secular basis. Some hospitals now hold a weekly memorial service in the hospital chapel for babies who have died before or after birth, with any recoverable ashes being scattered afterwards on a special plot set aside at the crematorium. Sadly, no ashes remain following cremation of miscarried babies, but many parents do still find cremation a helpful way of saying goodbye to their baby and a number of crematoriums are now willing to conduct such a service (see p. 99–101 for further details).

Events of birth and death in our society have been taken away from our homes and neighbourhoods and placed instead at a distance, in hospitals. Home births are still the exception, not the rule, and few of us ever see an adult's or child's dead body laid out at home any more because it all happens somewhere else. Of course death is painful and of course we want to shy away from anything associated with it, but death is also a reality and in pushing it away from ourselves as a community we are consequently denying ourselves many of the mourning rituals which could otherwise help us to cope and come to terms with what has happened. As it is, parents who want and need to accord their miscarried baby the ritual of a funeral and cremation or burial often have to face the embarrassment of family and friends who may well feel that they are over-reacting, going 'over the top' in some way, instead of recognizing that they are simply responding in a very natural and positive way to what has happened. What a curious society we are, that states that funeral rites are helpful and acceptable for a baby who dies after 28 weeks of gestation or more, but not for a baby who miscarries at 27 weeks or less. I find it frightening that society can exert pressures, however covertly, that are so great that they can over-ride natural human responses and force them to be suppressed, but then it is not so long ago that the public shame of producing an illegitimate baby often forced many young girls to abandon their newborn babies and leave them to die, against all natural instincts, and incredibly even in our so-called enlightened and permissive age, some girls still feel it necessary, because of the stigma attached, to conceal their pregnancies, give birth in secret and leave their babies to die from neglect at birth or else abandon them on the nearest hospital doorstep.

The black armbands and black and purple mourning clothes of Victorian times may seem excessive to us now, but they served a purpose. Anyone experiencing the acute vulnerability which follows a miscarriage might indeed welcome the return of a black armband which would say to others: 'I'm emotionally very raw just now, please treat me gently.'

Activities that may help

Amanda, whose twin daughters were miscarried at 23 weeks, later compiled a list of helpful activities based on replies from readers of the Miscarriage Association Newsletter, ranging from the physical, through the emotional to the spiritual. Understandably, heading the list came: 'It was vital to have a good cry and to be able to talk to someone about our losses'. The list included acts of comfort such as shared massage with aromatherapy oils, or 'putting my feet up with a cup of coffee, a sticky bun and a light-hearted novel' or 'a glass of wine and reading a magazine in a nice smelly hot bath'. It included physical activities such as a swim, singing or dancing to loud music within the privacy of home, or taking the dog for a walk. As Mana observed:

> Walking is good for the thought processes. Also it's good for the soul. You can cry in the park and blow your nose in the wind and no one will know the difference. And the dog makes me laugh – laughter is good medicine.

Creative activities were found to be helpful in restoring a sense of achievement and of being back in control, whether planting seeds or sewing patchwork quilts. Emotionally and spiritually, some women found comfort in writing down their experiences, others from reading relevant passages from the Bible such as Psalm 139 (138 in some versions), Isaiah 49, 1–5; Matthew 18, 1–11 and Corinthians 13. It is worth giving thought to any activities which you feel may help you to restore some rhythm and meaning to your life.

Relationships

Part of the process of reorganization and recovery involves adjusting to changes in personal relationships. Inevitably some will founder because you may find that you have needs which members of your family or existing friends can't or won't meet and also because you yourself will alter as a result of your experience of miscarriage. On the other hand, some relationships will deepen because of the experiences (see also Chapter 6). The emotional impact will inevitably affect your relationship with your partner and this is one of the consequences of miscarriage which I would like to talk about in the next chapter.

5

Coping As A Family

When miscarriage is perceived as a loss it becomes a death in the family and will affect all the members of the family to a greater or lesser degree.

The father

As I mentioned at the beginning of Chapter 3, not everyone will see the miscarriage as a loss, especially if it occurs very early on in pregnancy before he or she has formed any emotional attachment to the potential baby or made any emotional investment in the pregnancy; nor will couples necessarily respond in the same way. It would seem that most fathers feel that they have lost a potential, whereas most mothers feel that they have lost a reality. Again, much will depend on the stage of pregnancy reached when the miscarriage occurs. After our very early miscarriage, Pat and I both felt that we had lost a potential baby rather than an actual baby, but when our first daughter was miscarried at 27 weeks, Pat said that, even at that late stage, she was still only a potential baby to him because he had never known her, whereas I had felt her moving and responding inside me and therefore to me she was very real indeed.

Men have told me that their concern for their partner tends to over-ride their feelings about the unborn baby. Watching their partner in pain and in deep distress, even fearing that they may die when bleeding is heavy, are far more immediate and dominant emotions than the sense of intangible loss which may follow later.

Evidence suggests that men want not only to have children of their own but that also they want to provide their partners with the identity and role of mother. Part of the man's sense of loss, therefore, is likely to come from the unfulfilment of this aim. A baby serves as visible proof of the man's success in lovemaking and in giving his partner viable sperm. When pregnancy fails, some men find themselves wondering if their sperm was defective in some way, with the attendant feelings of guilt that this produces, and that they have 'failed' their partner. Alternatively, such is our natural need to blame ourselves that some men may feel that they have initiated a successful pregnancy only to sabotage it by indulging in lovemaking during the crucial months following conception and may feel afterwards that they should have abstained. As stressed before, lovemaking during pregnancy does not cause miscarriage. With the possible exception of certain very specific occasions (when a period would have been due or when a previous miscarriage occurred) lovemaking is safe at any time and in any position (though the increasing bulk of the baby may restrict the options as pregnancy progresses).

Many bereaved women turn to their partners for emotional support following a miscarriage and become very dependent on them for a while. This can be an added and difficult burden for the man when he is already trying to come to terms with his own grief. If the woman has always been very confident and competent, it can come as a shock to see her suddenly so lost and vulnerable and this is not only upsetting for the man, it can also be threatening to him if he has always relied on her strength and capability. He may find himself resenting her for being temporarily unable to cope and may experience very mixed emotions, wanting to comfort and support her but at the same time feeling angry with her for changing and angry with the situation that has made her change.

It is quite common for men to have ambivalent feelings towards the baby who has miscarried, on the one hand grieving for his or her death but on the other hand feeling angry towards the baby for causing such distress. This is natural, but again it can lead to unwarranted feelings of guilt.

Like women, many men find themselves having to cope with a host of mixed emotions following miscarriage. Much of what was said in Chapters 3 and 4 applies to bereaved fathers just as strongly as it does to bereaved mothers. Separating the chapters is not meant to imply that such grieving is exclusive in any way, simply that the reactions and responses are likely to differ in some respects because of the ways in which we see ourselves and our differing roles. Many men feel naturally protective towards their partners and consequently can feel very powerless at not preventing the miscarriage and of being unable to relieve their partner's pain at the time. Men have said to me how much they wish they could have taken on some of the physical pain themselves instead of having to stand by helplessly, watching their partner suffer. What they *can* do is offer support afterwards and because of this, many men consciously or unconsciously suppress or postpone their own grieving in order to be able to be strong for their partner. These men place their partner's needs above their own, sometimes at a high cost to themselves because sooner or later they, too, have to face and work through their own grief, and when it has been postponed this can be very difficult.

The most successful form of coping seems to arise when couples (again consciously or unconsciously) are able to take it in turns to grieve, alternately being the one to offer comfort or to be comforted. One woman who wrote to me said:

> My husband has been brilliant, he listens to me and is always there being supportive and understanding. I know I'm not fair to him at times with my moods . . . I do find it hard to be positive and not get depressed.

Balancing one's own needs and the needs of one's partner and family is not easy and much tolerance and understanding is required by all concerned. Ironically, men who suppress their grieving for their partner's sake can sometimes find themselves standing accused of being callous and unfeeling. Good communication is vital to avoid such misunderstandings and it is important therefore for men to express their feelings and not try to be strong all the time.

Some men find that there are very few openings for their own grief. This is especially likely to be true if they feel that they dare not place their jobs at risk by showing their distress at work and are equally reluctant to show their grief at home for fear of adding to their partner's distress. Well-meaning outsiders tend to ask, 'How's your poor wife?' instead of asking, 'How are you?'; as a result men can feel excluded and hurt, as well as feeling that they are being denied any entitlement to grieve.

Coping as a couple

A miscarriage may well be the first major crisis or loss which you have experienced together and inevitably both of you will alter as a result. Whether the miscarriage will draw you closer together or divide you apart will depend on how you both respond to it and how well you can express your feelings and share what is a very painful learning experience. If you misunderstand each other's needs or are unable to answer them, this can place great strain on the relationship. Couples who are unable to express and share their feelings may find that the miscarriage gives rise to other problems within their relationship. Conversely, when it fathoms the depths of love and caring which exist, it can strengthen the relationship and a very close bond can result.

The weeks following a miscarriage are inevitably very stressful and at such a time ordinary problems which would normally be manageable may loom very large and it can be difficult to keep a sense of perspective. It is also a time when priorities change and the focus shifts. Ambitions and goals which previously seemed important can suddenly seem pointless. This can lead to a sense of aimlessness, but it can also help to highlight the true priorities in life. Few couples who have experienced miscarriage ever take anything for granted again.

Just as women are likely to see pregnant women everywhere following their miscarriage, so, too, men may find themselves noticing far more than usual that there are prams in the street or children playing in the park. Such sights reinforce the loss of the parenthood that they should have been able to anticipate and enjoy and can leave them feeling cheated at a very deep level. Without being aware of it, depression can become a likely consequence for both partners and when it goes unrecognized in the relationship it can cause extra problems. As ever, talking about your feelings and being sensitive to the possibility of depression can help avert such problems.

Like bereaved mothers, fathers may also feel a strong need to find a cause, something to blame, and this can be a source of stress if they feel that their partner contributed to the miscarriage through something they did or did not do. They can find themselves feeling very angry with their partner but at the same time feeling guilty about such anger and as a result feeling obliged to suppress it. Their partner is likely to be blaming herself anyway, however un-warranted this may be, and if the man implies blame either overtly or covertly this is likely merely to compound his partner's feelings of guilt while at the same time making her feel hurt and angry with him for blaming her. The situation can be a very fraught one. If the temptation to attribute blame arises, it is worth reading all that is known about the possible causes of miscarriage, because this can help to reassure both of you that neither of you was to blame in any way.

Whilst it is understandable that if you have lost your baby, you may have an overwhelming need to have another as soon as possible, it is worth bearing in mind that, as every baby is unique, a new baby will not replace the one who has miscarried and will not necessarily remove depression and make everything seem right again. Indeed, if your grieving has not yet been resolved then a new baby may even increase your sense of depression. It is also worth remembering that, while both of you may be longing for another baby, one or both of you may feel that you cannot face going through such trauma again for a while.

Sometimes it is only when a woman suffers the devastating shock of a miscarriage that she becomes aware of just how much she wants a baby and she may find herself torn between the desire for another baby and the fear of another miscarriage. It can be very difficult for the man to understand the intense yearning for a subsequent baby which many women experience after a miscarriage. This craving may make her want to make love as a means to an end, not an end in itself, and the man can feel very used if he knows that his partner is only wanting to make love during the 'right' days of the month when conception is most likely.

Even if the woman is wanting another baby, the shock and grief of the miscarriage may cause a temporary loss of interest in sex, especially if she is still recovering from the effect of an ERPC or D and C operation. Feelings of being let down by her own body can also influence her response to lovemaking and she is likely to need reassurance and sensitivity in order to rebuild her self-confidence.

While for the woman the miscarriage may cause a loss of drive, for the man lovemaking may provide a vital physical release for pent-up emotions, but unless he can explain this need to his partner, she may resent him and feel: 'How can he possibly think about such a thing at a time like this?' It is important for couples to talk about their fears and their needs so that they are able to help each other as much as possible. While lovemaking can often suffer after a miscarriage, it can also be the most comforting act of all and can provide the deepest of bonds, linking the couple in a very profound awareness of sharing and consoling.

Coping as a single person

Occasionally relationships founder and couples separate just before or just after a miscarriage and then they find themselves having to cope with their loss without the help of a partner at home to offer comfort and support. This is also true where one partner is working away from home at the time and it can be the cause of added strain.

If there are older children or the responsibility of a job to consider, then the partner who is coping alone will have no opportunity to let go for a while. On the other hand if there are no other children and no job to maintain then life can feel very aimless and getting up in the mornings may prove increasingly difficult until a valid reason for doing so can be found.

It could be argued that at least those who are single can focus on their own needs during bereavement, without having to cope with the strain of trying to answer their partners' needs as well. They are free to express their grief when and how they wish, without fear of distressing or angering anyone else in the house, but this is of poor comfort to anyone needing love and support. Relatives and friends should be sensitive to the fact that those coping on their own may well need extra contact and help to prevent them from feeling isolated and alone with their loss.

Partners who have separated just before or just after the miscarriage may already be feeling that the miscarriage is like the final blow, proof that their once loving relationship has died in every sense and it can therefore be an additional grief to bear. Their confidence and self-esteem will have been damaged both by the miscarriage and by whatever has caused their relationship to end and therefore the time when they most need to go out, meet people and perhaps apply for a job is likely to be the time when they feel least able to do so. Again, relatives and friends can do much to restore self-esteem and self-confidence and they have a vital role to play.

Grandparents and close relatives

A miscarriage in the family can affect would-be grandparents much more deeply than many people realize. They experience a double grief, for not only do they have to try to cope with the loss of their potential grandchild, they also have the pain of seeing their own adult child grieving for the baby who has miscarried. They may also find that their adult son or daughter becomes emotionally dependent on them again for a while, seeking support and reassurance which perhaps, because of age or ill-health, they no longer feel able to give. It can be very difficult for a grandmother to be thrust without warning back into her mothering and nurturing role, just when she is least expecting it and perhaps feels least able to cope with it.

Just as young couples need to know that they can have and rear a child successfully, so grandparents need to know that they've done so. The arrival of the first grandchild confirms to grandparents that their years of parenting have borne fruit in every sense, as well as granting them a form of immortality. Miscarriage cuts off this link with immortality at one blow and serves as a harsh reminder that death is a reality. The need for a grandchild can be very powerful, but it is important for would-be grandparents to resist the urge to pressurize their adult son or daughter to have a baby simply to answer their own needs. If a grandchild seems to be a long time in coming, it means either that the young couple have made a conscious decision to wait or that waiting has been imposed on them. Either way, that is very private territory indeed and trespassers have only themselves to blame if they find themselves being prosecuted as a result.

If grandparents know that miscarriage has taken place, then any help and support which they can offer will be deeply appreciated even if it is not always openly acknowledged. Miscarriage can bring mothers and daughters or mothers-in-law and daughters-in-law very close together, or it can drive them apart, depending on how sensitively the situation is handled. What would-be grandparents must avoid at all costs is the temptation to offer any advice, however well-meaning, which could be interpreted as criticism. To say: 'I knew you should have given up working full-time' will not help and is very likely to damage your relationship with your daughter or daughter-in-law, as will any sentence beginning: 'You young girls of today . . .'. What is needed is not criticism but validation and support. At such a vulnerable time, tactless remarks can cause lasting harm within the family. Miscarriage can act as a catalyst, bringing to the surface underlying family tensions and feuds and therefore all relatives need to be very careful about what they say and do, and very sensitive to what couples who have just experienced a miscarriage are likely to be feeling.

If family relationships are already strained, then sadly the miscarriage and the unanswered needs which follow may simply increase the distances which already exist. For couples who do discover that their closest relatives can't answer their needs, this can be very disillusioning and difficult to accept at the time, especially as it may seem to be launching them onto the road to true independence when they feel least able to travel it. Becoming independent is yet another painful learning experience to have to handle, but if handled successfully it can serve eventually to bring families closer together, on an equal footing.

Miscarriage can create barriers, but it can also help to break them down and if you are able to confide in relatives and find that they are able to respond in return and to help you, then all of you may benefit and become closer as a result. Sometimes, ironically, it is only after a crisis or a tragedy that family relationships are able to develop and deepen.

Other children in the family

When we miscarry it is very tempting to try to convince ourselves that our existing child or children will remain unaware that anything has happened, but this is unlikely to be the case. Even if our children did not know that we were pregnant and were absent at the time of the miscarriage, they are still bound to sense the resulting distress and grief and may feel very threatened and confused that they know something is wrong but don't know what it is. If you had not yet told your children about your pregnancy and do not feel able to tell them about your early miscarriage, then it may be enough to explain to them that you are feeling unwell but hope to be better soon; but do not underestimate your children's ability to sense that something has suddenly upset you very deeply and made you very sad. You will need to be very careful about what you say when they are within earshot; talking freely to your partner, relative or friend at an unguarded moment may leave your children feeling anxious and hurt at being excluded, and of course, even if you do manage to be tactful and discreet at all times, others may not be so successful.

Our daughter Rebecca did not know until she was nine years old that she'd had an older sister who had miscarried and died at birth. I had felt that there was no sense in burdening her with a sorrow which was ours, not hers, but having made the mistake of telling an adult who I then realized might be likely to say something to her, I found myself having to tell Rebecca without any prior warning or preparation. She was shocked, angry and somehow relieved, saying to me: 'I knew, I just knew I wasn't the first and that I'd had a sister!' Maybe she had sensed it intuitively, maybe one of us had said something within her hearing when we thought that she was too young to understand. With hindsight, I wish we'd told her from the beginning, so that her sister's place in our family would have seemed natural instead of a complete revelation to her. Nor do I learn from experience, because when I found that I was able to 'pass off' my early miscarriage as backache I succumbed to the temptation to do so. Rebecca was only nine and Mary was only three. They had just recently learnt that they had lost an older sister and I did not want them to have to cope with the news of losing a potential younger brother or sister as well. The time passed and all seemed well until I decided to write this book and explained to a friend why I felt entitled to do so, having experienced both late and early miscarriage myself. 'I never knew you'd had an early miscarriage', said Rebecca in a very accusing voice and of course that was true. In trying to spare her I'd yet again excluded her and understandably she felt hurt as a result.

It is natural to want to spare our children from pain, but in doing so we may unintentionally create other problems for them and therefore honesty does seem to be the best policy. Obviously what we say to our children will depend on their ages and levels of understanding as well as on the stage of pregnancy reached at the time of the miscarriage. Early pregnancies will not necessarily have been apparent to them, whereas by a later stage they are likely to have noticed how their mother's shape has changed, to have talked about the awaited baby and formed their own images about the baby and plans for the future.

Whatever you do decide to tell your children, keep it simple and make it clear. It can be difficult enough trying to visualize a baby growing inside your mummy without then having to accept the reality that the baby is no longer there.

Children can be deeply affected by their mother's miscarriage because not only does it prove that there are no guarantees but it may also reveal that the parents they thought were all-powerful are in fact very vulnerable and both of these revelations can undermine their security. Even at such a difficult time it is important for parents, relatives and friends to make daily life as structured and as regular as possible in order to try and restore some of this damaged security. It is also important to emphasize that the doctor or hospital staff who attended the miscarriage did all that was possible to save the baby, to prevent any risk of children distrusting or fearing medical help in the future.

Children will need to be comforted both at the time and afterwards. This can be difficult for parents who are grieving but the best course of action is to talk to your children about your grief and to give them permission to grieve, too. Children who cannot express their feelings in language will express it in their behaviour. Young children may regress to a more infantile stage and most children are likely to seem especially demanding and difficult just when you most need them to behave well and take some of the pressure away from you, not add to it. If you can be aware that this is a natural reaction, it may help you to cope. Some children may become withdrawn and be 'too good', others may show their anger at what has happened by aggression towards you or others around them. If you can, try and defuse and channel such aggression. Tearing up cardboard boxes can be very therapeutic (I've done it myself at times and I can recommend it!). Encouraging your children to assist you through physical activities such as vacuuming, sweeping the yard or washing the car can also help, and such activities have the added bonus of making your children feel useful and valued, which is important to them at such a time.

To your children the miscarried baby may seem more like the loss of a potential than a reality, but even so they will be emotionally affected by what has happened and may show this in physical reactions, by developing new conditions or exacerbating existing ones such as asthma, eczema or hay fever. The more you can encourage your children to express their feelings, the less likely they are to develop physical reactions to the situation. Try and make time to talk and to listen to them, and encourage them to express themselves through writing, drawing, painting – even acting if this is possible. Where miscarriage has a major effect on the family, existing children are likely to find themselves trying to cope with mixed emotions of grief, anger, guilt and fear. These emotions need to be sanctioned by the parents as natural and given permission to surface and be worked through, otherwise there is a danger that they will be suppressed and cause problems later. It is now known that children, no matter how young, do feel grief both for their parents and for themselves when there is a loss in the family. They can feel intensely angry at what has happened and may want to blame either their parents or even themselves if they were feeling at all ambivalent about the awaited baby. Jealousy at the thought of having to share their parents with a new brother or sister is a very natural emotion, but it can lead to deep feelings of guilt if the baby then miscarries. Fear is likely to be present as well, because of the loss of security which accompanies a miscarriage, and the fear may express itself in new and seemingly irrational phobias about insects, spiders, certain noises or, very commonly, the dark. If parents can be aware of such potential reactions, then this may help them to offer reassurance and to be patient and understanding with their children, no matter how ridiculous or infuriating the new and unexpected phobias may seem to be at the time.

The two key words in coping as a family after a miscarriage seem to be honesty and understanding: honesty about your own feelings; understanding about the feelings of others. When these are kept in mind and the consequences of miscarriage worked through together, with tolerance and sensitivity to the needs of all concerned, then families can emerge not just intact but strengthened and more united than ever by their shared experience.

Relatives have a crucial role to play. Whilst the next chapter is intended to guide friends and colleagues as to how best to offer support, what applies to them applies equally to relatives, so for those who want to know what to say or do (or avoid saying and doing) when someone in their family experiences miscarriage, I hope the following chapter will be of assistance.

6

Who Can Help?

It's strange how planning and writing this book has helped me to recognize some wrong assumptions. I had always assumed that the intense pain that I felt over our first daughter's death meant that I had grieved fully for her and I now know that there was a great deal of unresolved grief still inside me, waiting to be acknowledged and worked through. I had also assumed that, since it is now 17 years since she miscarried, nearly 12 years since Elizabeth died in a cot death and 7 years since I had the early miscarriage, such a long time gap might be too long, allowing me to forget some of the immediacy and intensity of the grief that follows the sudden and unexpected death of a much-wanted baby, whether from cot death after birth or miscarriage before birth. Wrong again. I was thinking about how the years have passed, sitting in this quiet Welsh cottage, listening to the rain hurling itself against the window and Radio 4 telling me about today's papers, when I heard the broadcaster say: 'Most of today's papers carry coverage of the death yesterday of Anne Diamond's four-month-old baby, a victim of cot death' and straightaway I was back there again, weeping for Anne and her family and for all those thousands of other families who have known the tragedy of cot death, and for myself, for a pain that never goes away. The years between have seen me change, adapt, hopefully even grow in mind and spirit, but any fears that I might have become too distant to remember the pain of loss vanished with that announcement. Anne Diamond is a well-known name and face because of her years on television as presenter on TV-am. Two years earlier she had come to our fund-raising James Bond première, helping to raise money for research into cot death. I have always stressed to everyone that cot death is not infectious, that you can't 'catch it' in some way by reading about it or taking an interest in it. Now here was Anne, suddenly facing a tragedy which she had actively tried to prevent. The irony was too much and so I wept and heard myself saying to the empty room: 'I'm so sorry, so very sorry'; it hit me then that ultimately that's the best we can do when someone suffers a deep loss. If someone known to you has just had a miscarriage, there's no point in trying to explain it or justify it or search for a way to reduce or minimize what has happened. What you can say, to express your own feelings and give her permission to express hers, is simply to say: 'I'm so sorry', and to be sensitive as to whether she then requires privacy or a good listener, and to be willing to offer which ever she needs at the time.

The Compassionate Friends, an organization of bereaved parents, has published a very valuable list of DOs and DON'TS to guide people about helpful and unhelpful reactions following the death of a baby or child. As so much of it is also applicable to miscarriage, I thought it might be helpful to include the relevant sections here:

DOs

- DO let your genuine concern and caring show.
- DO be available . . . to listen, to run errands, to help with the other children, or whatever else seems needed at the time.
- DO say you are sorry about what happened and about their pain.
- DO allow them to express as much grief as they are feeling at the moment and are willing to share.
- DO encourage them to be patient with themselves, not to expect too much of themselves and not to impose any 'shoulds' on themselves.
- DO allow them to talk about the child they have lost as much and as often as they want to.
- DO give special attention to brothers and sisters (they too are hurt and confused and in need of attention

DON'Ts

- DON'T let your own sense of helplessness keep you from reaching out to a bereaved parent.
- DON'T avoid them because you are uncomfortable (being avoided by friends adds pain to an already intolerably painful experience).
- DON'T say how you know how they feel (unless you've lost a child yourself you probably don't know how they feel).
- DON'T say 'You ought to be feeling better by now' or anything else which implies a judgement about their feelings.
- DON'T tell them what they *should* feel or do.
- DON'T change the subject when they mention their dead child.
- DON'T avoid mentioning the child out of fear of reminding them of their pain

which their parents may not be able to give at this time).

(they haven't forgotten it!).

- DON'T try to find something positive (e.g. a moral lesson, closer family ties, etc.) about the child's death.

- DON'T point out at least they have their other children (children are not interchangeable, they cannot replace each other).

- DON'T say that they can always have another child (even if they wanted to and could, another child would not replace the child they've lost).

- DON'T suggest that they should be grateful for their other children (grief over the loss of one child does not discount parent's love and appreciation of their living children).

Prepared by Lee Schmidt, Parent Bereavement Outreach, Santa Monica, California, and reproduced by courtesy of the Compassionate Friends.

Often friends are only too willing to help but feel totally at a loss as to how to do so. They can help in a practical way, of course, by cooking meals and doing the washing or the shopping, but they can also help in an emotional way, by giving bereaved families the openings they need in order to talk about what has happened. It takes a true and brave friend to do this and I have heard of people crossing the road to avoid someone who has just had a miscarriage, not as a form of rejection or implied blame but simply because they did not know what to say. Most take the easy option and talk about everything but the miscarriage, even though it will be silently dominating every conversation.

For friends to be of help to you after your miscarriage, you will need to be very honest about your feelings yourself. Friends will be so afraid of unintentionally upsetting you that it will be up to you to guide them as to whether you want to talk about your miscarriage or avoid talking about it on any particular day. Don't try to 'spare' either yourself or your friends because it can't be done. Miscarriage is a shared loss, it affects our friends as well as ourselves. At least, by speaking of your feelings of sadness you will be giving your friends permission to speak of their feelings as well.

Friends can be both the most helpful and the least helpful people following a miscarriage. Most helpful, if they are willing to listen and especially if they have had their own experience of miscarriage and can therefore understand even more so, perhaps, than husbands, partners or relatives exactly what you are experiencing and feeling at the time; least helpful, if they fail to understand or to make themselves available, or if they make thoughtless and hurtful remarks, like the ones made to Amanda:

It'll be much easier to finish the thesis now you've lost the twins.

You would never have coped with them anyway.

You wouldn't have wanted a handicapped baby. (They weren't.)

How do you know what sex they were? Did you actually see them?

Now you two can have some fun.

You must go travelling before you start again.

You're young yet . . . plenty of time.

I have already mentioned in Chapter 4 that friendships will alter as a consequence of miscarriage, some faltering, some deepening. As a friend, try to ensure that it is the latter which takes place – be caring, tactful and available. One way of ensuring this is to avoid common traps:

(1)   The urge to encourage your bereaved friend to 'get back to normal' as quickly as possible, because this minimizes her loss. If you praise your friend for coping so well, in the hope that she will find this helpful, the likelihood is that she will hear instead the risk of future criticism if she fails to cope, and this may merely add to the strain which she is already feeling.

(2)   The temptation to minimize the effect of the miscarriage by suggesting that your friend or relative will soon forget – she won't. One woman who wrote to me had to endure her mother-in-law saying: 'You'll have forgotten all about it in a few weeks.' Another wrote: 'I thought at times I couldn't possibly have any tears left . . . I'll never forget the experience. I don't want to forget it.'

(3)   The temptation to minimize the effect of the miscarriage by suggesting that your friend can soon have another baby. This is a point made by the Compassionate Friends and it is an important one. Even if your friend can and does have a subsequent baby this will in no way reduce her sense of loss after her miscarriage. Babies are not interchangeable and they are not replaceable. To say, as so many older people do: 'Oh, you're young and healthy, you'll soon have another' is totally inappropriate and unhelpful. It would be better to give bereaved couples open permission to acknowledge and grieve for the baby they have lost.

(4)   The temptation to suggest possible causes. Someone who has just had a miscarriage will already be searching around for sticks with which to beat herself, she does not need to be handed any more from you! If you have constructive knowledge about known and recognized causes of miscarriage, by all means offer to share this knowledge, but keep private theories to yourself because they are more likely to do harm than good.

(5)   The temptation to reduce or withdraw your support after a while on the assumption that all is well. The natural tendency is for friends to descend, sometimes in large numbers, soon after the miscarriage, at a time when peace and privacy may in fact be what is needed most, and then to let their support dwindle after a short while because the person who has had the miscarriage appears to be coping. If possible, try to co-ordinate with other friends to avoid the risk of such 'feasts and famines' and to ensure that support is always available. It is well recognized that three months after a bereavement can be an especially difficult time, because having made some initial progress the bereaved person may suddenly feel that she is slipping back and making no progress at all. It is then that she may need support most. What has happened is that, after original high expectations of herself, she is having to adjust to the realities involved in grieving and to accept that, for most of us, it is not a sprint, it is a marathon.

(6)   The temptation, as soon as a subsequent pregnancy is announced, to assume that a new baby will heal all the hurt and

make everyone happy again. It won't, and your friend will need support throughout the subsequent pregnancy to allay fears and anxieties which are an almost inevitable consequence of miscarriage. Don't be afraid to mention the previous miscarriage while your friend is pregnant – the one guarantee you can have is that she won't have forgotten. Speaking about it can give her a much-needed opening to talk about her memories of the past and her fears and hopes for the future.

Having given a somewhat daunting list of traps to avoid, here are three positive actions which you can take to help your friend following her miscarriage.

(A)   Acknowledge its existence, talk about it and allow her to talk about it, too. I know I've already mentioned this, but it can't be stressed too often. Miscarriage is still largely seen as a taboo subject. You can help to break that taboo. I called this book *Talking about Miscarriage* because that is what needs to be done. There is still a conspiracy of silence surrounding miscarriage, an implication that it is an unacceptable event which must be kept hidden. Of the women who wrote to me, most apologized for 'rambling on' about their miscarriage but added that it was such a relief and comfort to have an opportunity to write about it. Why apologize? Maybe we're too brave for our own good. What we ourselves perceive as 'rambling on' is in fact a perfectly natural and justified response to our experience and loss, yet we find ourselves having to cope not only with our loss but also with the unacceptable face of miscarriage. Amanda wrote:

> Sometimes we were invited to occasions where other guests were pregnant or had brand-new babies. On such occasions we would have to pretend we had never had children – deny our daughters had ever existed . . . Once I wrecked a smart dinner party by bursting into tears when the hostess started to speculate on the likelihood of another guest having a twin pregnancy.

Many women wrote to me of their deep distress when subjected to other pregnant women talking endlessly of their pregnancies, oblivious to the one which ended in miscarriage, as if denying that it ever existed or implying that it ought to be forgotten.

> The girls at work . . . would all be chatting about their pregnancies, antenatal etc. and I'd sit quietly wanting to die.

Maybe we shouldn't sit quietly; maybe in the face of such insensitivity we should declare how we are truly feeling even if it does cause embarrassment; maybe seeking open acknowledgement of miscarriage would help to give it the attention and understanding it warrants – but it would take a special kind of courage to do so, and I suspect that most of us will continue to opt for the kind of courage which makes us strive instead to go on sitting quietly and keeping all the suffering inside.

No wonder so many women think that they are an oddity, an embarrassing exception to the rules of pregnancy, because few of them know beforehand how common an occurrence miscarriage can be. Margaret Leroy, in her book *Miscarriage*, points out that miscarriage, like menstruation, involves a lot of bleeding from the vagina. She goes on to make the point that miscarriage thus brings together two of our most powerful taboos – death and menstruation – and says that this may help to explain why it remains such a hidden grief.

(B)   Allow your friend to mourn and encourage her to use any mourning rituals which she finds useful, because your acceptance and encouragement will help to validate them for her.

(C)   Be sensitive to the needs of everyone in the family. The natural tendency is to focus entirely on your friend because she is the one who has suffered the miscarriage, but her partner and any children in the family will also be grieving, so do give them some of your time and offer them the opportunity to talk about what has happened. Husbands and partners can feel very helpless and excluded following a miscarriage and children can feel very threatened by their parents' obvious distress, because it proves that they are not invincible. Children need to express their grief, too, and may want to comfort their parents without knowing best how to do so. By making yourself available to them, taking an interest in them and listening to them, you will be able to give them valuable openings to express their own fears and feelings.

Your doctor and hospital staff

Both the GP and the hospital staff have a very important role to play. What they say and do (or fail to do) will have a crucial impact on anyone experiencing a miscarriage and therefore the role of all medical staff, because it is so important, will be looked at in detail in the next chapter: How The Medical Profession Can Help. Whilst the

next chapter will be addressed primarily to health-care professionals, I am hoping that mothers (and indeed everyone affected by
miscarriage, including relatives and friends) will read the chapter
with a view to discovering how best to benefit from the medical help
which is available and how to encourage future improvements in the
care offered before, during and after a miscarriage.

Colleagues at work

If you were working at the time of your miscarriage, then two
decisions face you: (1) When to return to work, assuming that you
plan to do so, and (2) if the pregnancy had not been announced,
whether to tell your colleagues what has happened. Obviously, if
people at work already knew that you were pregnant, then you have
no choice but to acknowledge your miscarriage – if only to avoid the
risk of someone asking how the baby is progressing. Unfortunately,
telling everyone about the miscarriage and coping with the ensuing
sympathy (and sometimes lack of it) can be a considerable strain at a
time when you are still feeling so vulnerable. Miscarriage is a very
intimate event and therefore you may feel very awkward about
having to report it to someone senior who makes you feel shy at the
best of times. Quite often, colleagues will have been unaware that
you were pregnant. Some women are reluctant to mention their
condition precisely for that reason – that pregnancy is still seen by
some as a 'delicate condition' which will automatically make them a
liability and render them incapable at work. This same fear of being
thought incapable at work leads many women who concealed their
pregnancies to explain away their temporary absence at the time of
the miscarriage with the excuse of 'flu or a minor ailment. Doctors
often collude in this approach, offering to write something vague on
the sick note to avoid the necessity of mentioning miscarriage at all –
again, the suggestion that it is an embarrassment, something
shameful which must be hidden away and denied. Part of the
responsibility for this attitude, of course, must lie with ourselves,
those of us who have experienced miscarriage and yet chosen to
conceal the fact from our colleagues because to acknowledge it
seems like an admission of failure and an outside intrusion into a
very private event. In this respect, I have to plead guilty because
when I had to have two days away from my work as a playgroup
supervisor at the time of my early miscarriage, I gave the reason as
backache. It was true, I did suffer backache throughout the entire

event, but it was also a way of avoiding a sympathy which I knew I would find difficult to handle and also of avoiding a public announcement about a very private wish. After five years, we had decided to try for another baby, one I wanted very much. I did not want that desire to be generally known, with everyone watching my outline every month for signs of success. The fear of potential failure was too great. The immediate conception had given my confidence a wonderful boost, but the early miscarriage which followed it had dealt me a crushing blow. Back came all my instincts to creep away and hide somewhere (no wonder my star sign is Cancer the Crab, I seem to spend much of my time wanting to retreat and hide in my shell!). The last thing I wanted was to feel exposed to public view and sympathy, so I kept up the excuse of backache and blushed with shame when one kind colleague at work offered to lend me her heat lamp as a remedy.

I was wrong to conceal my miscarriage, I know that now because I know from experience that the most unexpected people can prove to be the most understanding and helpful. I should have had more faith in those around me instead of deliberately keeping them at a distance, thereby depriving myself of much potential support. But I like my shell, it's safe in there and venturing out from it makes me feel exposed and vulnerable, so I do genuinely sympathize with anyone else who experiences a miscarriage but who finds it very difficult to acknowledge that experience to others.

When to return to work is a decision which only you should make. Physically you may recover quite quickly and seem to your doctor to be perfectly fit for work, but only you can assess how much the emotional impact is affecting you. Returning to work too soon is likely to do more harm than good, so don't try and force yourself before you feel ready to cope. Be prepared for the likelihood that you may experience feelings of intense vulnerability and weepiness at times when you do go back to work. There may well be other women at your workplace who are pregnant and you will have to face them and accept them every time you walk through the door. There will be some colleagues who will embarrass you with their sympathy, others who will upset you by their indifference. Until you feel strong enough to handle your own emotions and the behaviour of others, do not attempt to return no matter how much you feel you should be doing so.

Being at home if you are used to being at work can make you feel very lost and disorientated. Being back at work can help, giving you company and keeping you busy, but unfortunately work may not seem the same any more. The depth and intensity of the experience of birth and death which you have just undergone may make work suddenly seem a pointless and irrelevant exercise now, and though these feelings may be only temporary, they can make it very difficult to cope and carry on as before. On the other hand, working may give you a sense of purpose and restore some of your damaged self-confidence (provided you do not return before you feel ready to do so, since finding it difficult to cope will merely undermine your confidence still further). Anyone financially dependent on their work will feel very torn between the need to earn and the fear of being unable to cope so soon after the miscarriage. For those who had been planning to leave in readiness for the baby, a major psychological adjustment will be needed since the future you had been visualizing has died with the baby. Even if you are able to maintain or reclaim your current position at work, in some ways this will simply reinforce the finality of the miscarriage and this can be hard to bear.

If colleagues can be aware of all the stresses and mixed emotions which those who have just had a miscarriage are likely to be feeling, then hopefully they will be able to help by respecting such feelings, being tactful in their approach and keeping any additional work stresses to a minimum. It is not an easy time for anyone, but handled well, the experience of miscarriage can convert colleagues into friends, and close and lasting bonds at work can result, to the benefit of everyone.

Support groups

Of all the various forms of support available, the most valuable can often come from your local support group of the Miscarriage Association. This is because those who run such groups have been there, they know what it's like, they understand what you're saying and what you're feeling and they will allow you to talk freely. They won't patronize, they won't swamp you with horror stories to outmatch your own trauma, they will simply listen and share and help you to cope. You may arrive feeling an awkward newcomer, not knowing what to expect, and in time find that you want to help run such a group yourself, taking over as others follow the natural pattern of recovering and moving on once their needs have been met. Being involved in such a group is not a commitment for life (unless you want it to be so) but it can be a good way of doing something positive, taking action by reaching out to others and allowing them to reach out to you. When your miscarriage occurs without an explanation and seems so senseless, making everything else seem pointless as well, then helping to fund-raise for research into the causes and prevention of miscarriage can make you feel that you are achieving something, doing something tangible and positive to help prevent others from ever experiencing what you have had to go through.

Local groups are linked to the Miscarriage Association but they are run on a voluntary basis by women who have one important factor in common – they all know the heartache of miscarriage. They may come from widely differing backgrounds and their miscarriages may have been early or late, single or repeated, recent or a number of years ago, but they will know how you are feeling and will be able to give you accurate information and valuable support, both after your miscarriage and during any subsequent pregnancy. Local groups of the National Childbirth Trust (NCT) and Birthright are also often able to give good support, and other groups exist which may be able to answer your specific needs, such as SATFA (Support After Termination for Fetal Abnormality) and the Stitch Network (for anyone who has been diagnosed as having an incompetent cervix). Addresses for groups such as these can be found at the end of the book.

Counsellors

If you feel that you are in need of professional counselling, do ask your doctor for a referral or consult Yellow Pages (under 'Psychotherapy and analysis' or 'Therapists'). The addresses and telephone numbers of the British Association of Counselling, and the British Association of Psychotherapists are given at the end of this book. Your Health Visitor, Social Services Department or Adult Education Centre may also be able to recommend a counsellor, and your local support group of the Miscarriage Association may have knowledge of someone who has helped in the past. It is important to talk about your loss and if you find it easier to talk to an independent and objective stranger rather than someone you know, then counselling may be the answer – either for you as an individual or for you both as a couple, if you are finding it difficult to talk to each other about your feelings or to understand each other's needs at the time.

Psychotherapy can also be of help to anyone coping with the trauma of miscarriage. The term 'psychotherapy' is sometimes off-putting because of its similarity to psychiatry, which for many people still implies that mental instability is involved. Try to remember that your responses to your miscarriage are natural. Psychotherapists are highly skilled in helping people to talk through their problems and to understand what they are feeling and why, so don't be deterred by the name.

Hospital social workers are another potential source of help, so if your miscarriage takes place in hospital you would be fully entitled to ask to see a hospital social worker if you feel that he or she might be able to help.

The clergy

Having a miscarriage can make us rethink our whole attitude to God and, as mentioned in Chapter 4, we may find ourselves either turning towards him or alternatively pulling away and rejecting God because of what has happened. We tend to assume that if we are not regular church attenders, then we are not 'entitled' to contact our local minister of religion for help, but this is not the case. Ministers of all denominations have wide knowledge and experience of the effects of bereavement because of their parish work, and can often give great comfort – as well as offering help and insight to anyone struggling to understand what it's all about. It's hard enough trying to grasp the 'meaning of life' at the best of times, let alone when life seems to have no meaning at all. Don't automatically reject your local minister out of hand as a source of help, for he won't reject you and may prove very helpful. This is true also of hospital chaplains, so if your miscarriage takes place in hospital it is worth asking to see the chaplain if you feel that he might be able to help.

Books, magazine articles and media coverage

When you have just had a miscarriage you will not only be acutely aware of every pregnant woman in the vicinity, you will also find that any article on miscarriage in a newspaper or magazine will leap from the page at you, regardless of whether you want to ignore it or read it avidly for any information you can glean. There are many more pregnant women than there are items about miscarriage! The fact that it is still largely a hidden subject may help to explain why there are no accurate statistics about its incidence and frequency, but at least the situation is improving. There are now some very good books on the subject (I have listed these at the end of this book) and magazine articles are beginning to appear. But there is still a long way to go. Perhaps those who plan radio and television programmes and edit magazines do not realize that there is such a need waiting to be met. If we can voice our needs and make them known, we will increase the chance that programme and magazine editors will hear and respond.

7

How The Medical Profession
Can Help

I have to admit that I found myself approaching this chapter with some trepidation, aware that I had no wish to alienate those many members of the medical profession who do their best to help women experiencing miscarriage but aware, too, that many of these women have needs which are not being met and which, with a change in attitude rather than resources, could be met more successfully in the future. In writing what follows, I realize that I am really addressing two distinct groups of people: first, the health-care professionals, in the hope that as a result they will feel able to answer more closely the needs of mothers experiencing miscarriage, and second, the mothers themselves, in the hope that they will become better informed about best practice and possible problems and therefore better enabled to ask for and obtain appropriate consideration and treatment.

One of the harsh realities which those of us who experience miscarriage have to recognize and accept is that often, when miscarriage threatens, there is very little that doctors can do to prevent the miscarriage from taking place. It is a very difficult situation because the women concerned are likely to feel that doctors are failing them by not doing anything, and the doctors concerned are likely to feel that such women are being unrealistic by having expectations which cannot be met. Doctors, midwives and nurses are trained to be active, to 'do something', and miscarriage often faces them with a situation where there is nothing that can be done. This can be very frustrating and undermining for them. If intervention could save the pregnancy, most doctors would be only too happy to intervene. Miscarriage is distressing not only for the women concerned but also for the doctors and members of the medical staff as well. It is understandable that some doctors and nurses feel the need to use detachment not just as a means of maintaining efficiency but also as a form of self-protection against the pain and distress involved, but, as anyone who has experienced miscarriage will verify, there is, too, an overwhelming need for them to balance this with care and concern. Most do care – what is needed is for their patients to see that they care.

Before the miscarriage

Your family doctor

Family doctors have a vital role to play before, during and after miscarriage. An appropriate response will always be remembered and appreciated. An inappropriate response will never be forgotten or forgiven.

Every month, women bleed. Once menstruation is well established, our monthly periods hold few surprises. Sometimes there can be considerable loss of blood, but we are able to accept this as a natural part of our womanhood and we can cope. What doctors (and partners) can easily underestimate is the intense shock and fear which can accompany unexpected bleeding. The nearest equivalent would be for men to try and ask themselves how they would react if they paid a routine visit to the toilet and suddenly found themselves passing blood, possibly a copious amount of blood. A man passing blood unexpectedly would fear for himself. A pregnant woman passing blood unexpectedly has to cope with fear not only for herself but also for her unborn child. Understandably any woman finding herself in this situation is likely to want to contact her doctor as soon as possible, for reassurance and an accurate diagnosis. A sympathetic and appropriate response to her call for help is essential. It is not the time to be blocked by the receptionist or given vague advice by her doctor over the telephone to 'go and rest'. Some may be able to cope, but most will need to be seen and diagnosed to try and discover the cause of the bleeding, with the offer of a subsequent ultrasound scan, if appropriate. Even though, as the family doctor, you may feel that there is nothing useful that you can do at this stage, your presence itself is important and the information which you can give concerning bleeding in pregnancy and concerning potential miscarriage can be invaluable. Forewarned *is* forearmed. Your role is not to try and protect your patient from what may be going to happen but to be truthful and informative. Imagination and nightmares can often be worse than reality anyway. A woman who has been prepared for what may happen will be in a much better position to cope if it does, and will have been spared the added pain of false illusions.

There is a natural but usually wrong assumption among those of us who are threatened with miscarriage that going to hospital means something can and will be done to save the pregnancy. Since we are brought up to believe that hospitals exist to make people better, disillusion and disappointment can result when this fails to be the case and miscarriage ensues. A practical forewarning by you as the family doctor can help us to avoid building up any unrealistic expectations.

Hospital staff

From my contact with women who have miscarried, the impression I receive is that most are very willing to recognize the restrictions imposed by lack of Health Service funding. What they find far more difficult to accept is the apparent lack of care or compassion on the part of some members of hospital medical or nursing staff. Ironically, the care and compassion are usually there but often they are not outwardly shown. What is needed is for staff to allow themselves to be more open and communicative, so that women who miscarry can see that most doctors and nurses *do* care and *do* feel compassion for them in their loss.

What ward?

Again, Health Service restrictions will inevitably play a part in determining what facilities can be offered to women threatened with or experiencing miscarriage, but within these restrictions the most important factor is that these women should be welcomed, reassured and made to feel that they belong and have a right to be within the hospital, instead of feeling, as many do, that they should be issued with a bell and a sign to confirm the impression given that they are somehow 'unclean'. Busy hospitals are likely to have at least four miscarrying patients at any one time. This is a significant number and yet many women state that they are made to feel like misfits and find themselves shunted from ward to ward instead of being cared for in an appropriate way.

For many women, the first contact with their hospital is via the casualty department, where they are likely to encounter a long wait and lack of privacy. It is all too easy for such women, queuing for attention in the crowded and busy casualty department, to feel out of place and ignored, if not totally abandoned when they are most in need of attention and reassurance. Miscarriage is distressing enough within the privacy of one's own home, let alone a crowded waiting room, yet, as I mentioned in Chapter 2, women have told me that they have been made to wait on chairs or stretcher trolleys in full view, in well-advanced premature labour, where their greatest fear was of bleeding copiously and publicly all over the floor. Even allowing for lack of facilities this is a situation which should never, ever, arise. If possible, it is usually less traumatic for a woman who may be miscarrying to be admitted straight to a ward via her family doctor. If she is still in early pregnancy then she is likely to be admitted to a gynaecology or emergency ward. If her pregnancy is advanced, she will probably be admitted to a maternity ward. Sometimes she is simply placed wherever there happens to be a spare bed, no matter how inappropriate to her needs this may be. There is no ideal: on a gynaecology ward she is likely to encounter women who are having terminations or undergoing sterilization or hysterectomy, having decided to postpone or end their childbearing while she is being thwarted of her chance to begin or continue her own childbearing time; on an emergency ward she will be spared such contact but will encounter staff who are geared to coping with medical emergencies rather than the needs created by miscarriage; on a maternity or postnatal ward she is likely to be within sight and hearing of pregnant women and newborn babies, which can be heart-breaking.

When our daughter miscarried, I was returned afterwards to a side-room adjoining a large and very busy ward filled with canned pop music, the chatter of mothers and the cries of newborn babies. Any hopes that my little side-room would afford me some peace and privacy were soon dashed. The pop music played relentlessly and the two hit songs which were being 'plugged' incessantly at the time can even now, 17 years later, still send shivers down my spine when I hear them on the radio. So that they could check on me when passing, the nurses insisted on my door remaining open. Perhaps a relevant notice might have protected me from the heavily pregnant young girl who soon came in, sat down, and, pressing her nightdress tightly against her outline, insisted on showing me how much her baby was moving inside her when my own baby had just died. I suppose such an encounter had its uses because I can remember thinking: 'If I can endure this then I can endure anything', but it was neither kind nor necessary.

Where it is possible to set aside a small ward especially for women threatened with or experiencing miscarriage, the staff are much more likely to be geared to their special needs and patients will be able to draw comfort and support from each other. Obviously in some hospitals this will not be possible, but when a woman is admitted because of miscarriage, it can help if staff explain why she is being placed wherever she does find herself placed. Letting her know that they are offering her the best they can within the restrictions of the Health Service and similarly, giving her information and preparation concerning the possible courses of action which may be taken (including none, if this is appropriate) will at least make her feel that thought and consideration have been given to her situation.

Health visitors, community midwives and antenatal staff

As several mothers have pointed out, it seems ironic that usually contact is not made until the most critical stage of pregnancy has already passed – in other words, those all-important first few weeks when the baby is forming, so it can be of great help if health visitors and community midwives make contact and offer support as soon as the pregnancy is confirmed. It would also help if mothers could be notified at the time of their previous miscarriage if such support in any future pregnancy might be available.

More and more we are becoming aware of just how vulnerable the fetus can be during the early weeks of development and many women are paying increased attention to their lifestyles during pregnancy, and trying to ensure a healthy diet to promote a healthy pregnancy, avoiding anything such as smoking, alcohol or drugs (including over-the-counter medicines such as paracetamol) which may have an adverse effect. Having asked a pharmacist for guidance about the use of over-the-counter medicines during pregnancy, the advice is firm: avoid *all* medicines, including apparently innocuous preparations such as throat lozenges or cough remedies. If you feel you must take something then consult your doctor first. Awareness has been heightened by better publicity and by the existence of organizations such as Birthright, Foresight and the National Childbirth Trust that work so hard to ensure that every potential baby is given the best possible chance of survival and good health. Inevitably, however, there will be mothers who take the greatest care during pregnancy and yet experience miscarriage or stillbirth. They are bound to know of others who continue to smoke and drink throughout pregnancy and to neglect their own health and that of their unborn child and yet who still succeed in producing full-term, healthy, beautiful babies.

Health visitors, like doctors, have done much to ensure that mothers known to them are immune to rubella, the mild infection of German measles which can be so devastating to the developing baby if contracted in early pregnancy. If possible, health visitors already in contact with mothers of young children should be sensitive to possible warning signs if one of their mothers contacts them for advice during pregnancy. Very often mothers feel able to consult their health visitor or practice nurse rather than their doctor. Even though they may be very worried about unexpected and un-explained symptoms, they may still feel that: 'Oh, I don't like to bother the doctor' and will turn to the health visitor or nurse for reassurance or advice. Listening carefully to their symptoms and giving the right advice at this stage (including referral to the doctor, if necessary) may help to prevent miscarriage at a later stage. Similarly, community midwives who have already attended mothers during previous pregnancies can be invaluable during subsequent pregnancies, especially if these take place following a miscarriage. Often they will not need to 'do' anything, their presence and support will be enough to allay any fears. Since it seems likely that stress can have an influence on the developing baby, anything which promotes peace of mind in the mother is likely to benefit all concerned.

As antenatal staff are only too well aware, many mothers do not even realize that they are pregnant until the pregnancy is well established and the first few weeks have passed. Hospital antenatal care can only begin once the mother has been referred by her doctor, and the time which can be given to each mother is restricted by the pressures under which antenatal staff have to work and the sheer number of mothers waiting to be seen. But even within these limitations, staff can do much to enhance or detract from the quality of each pregnancy. It is very difficult for staff always to remember that what is so monotonously routine for them may be totally new for the mother concerned. Expectant mothers need staff who will listen, care and respond. A doctor or midwife who waits until he or she is leaving the room before asking abruptly: 'Any problems?' is of no help to the mother who may have very genuine worries, some of which may be trivial and easily allayed, others of which could be the forewarning of something serious. A knowledgeable member of staff who is willing to listen may well succeed in detecting a potential problem and preventing future complications. At the risk of stating the obvious, staff need to be constantly alert to possible danger signs and to ask the right questions at the right time.

For any woman whose baby has died either before or after birth, returning to the same clinic for her next pregnancy is a very emotional experience and she is likely to feel distressed and vulnerable. It is essential for staff to familiarize themselves with the mother's notes beforehand if careless blunders are to be avoided. Recounting one's obstetric history may be necessary, but doing so · can touch some very raw nerves indeed. Perhaps a star or mark on the file could be used to alert staff immediately to the fact that there has been a previous tragedy. Mothers need acknowledgement of their previous baby or babies and it can help greatly if staff are able to raise the subject in a way which shows that they care, rather than by ignoring what has happened or obliging the mother to raise the subject herself. Clinic appointments for mothers who have experienced bereavement are bound to be stressful, but staff who do what they can to help will always be remembered afterwards with gratitude.

During the miscarriage

The family doctor

Most doctors tend to see their patients either before or after the miscarriage has occurred, but if you, the family doctor, are asked to visit while the miscarriage is actually taking place, then your presence can do much to reassure your patient and help her to cope with what is happening. Yes, it's messy and yes, it's distressing, but a woman who is miscarrying needs attention just as much, if not more than, a woman in full-term labour and it is not the time for distance or detachment. One woman, who miscarried at 9 weeks, described to me what happened when she asked her doctor to visit:

> A locum came. He stood at the bedroom door, wearing a suit and a mac. He never even took his mac off.

Going into labour for the first time is by definition a new and therefore potentially frightening experience. Full-term labour carries with it the excitement and anticipation of the long-awaited baby. Labour preceding miscarriage places the woman in the worst possible situation, with her body disobeying her deepest wishes and expelling the not-yet-completed baby she so wants to keep inside. Added to the physical trauma of the labour itself is the emotional trauma resulting from the awareness that there is to be no happy outcome, so it is scarcely surprising that such a woman should feel the need for someone with skill, knowledge and authority – be it doctor or midwife – to reassure her, offer her appropriate pain relief and help her through the experience.

Depending on the reason for the miscarriage and the stage of pregnancy reached, there may well be a recognizable fetus at the end of the labour and the mother will need sensitive practical advice on what to do with this tiny, potential baby who has left her body despite all the love she was wanting to give. To suggest: 'Oh, just flush it down the loo' may be practical but it is crass in the extreme and takes no account of the emotional investment of the parents. It would be more appropriate to try and find out the parents' feelings first and then advise accordingly. The parents may be hoping that the fetus will be examined and tests done to try and establish the cause of the miscarriage. Since tests are not usually carried out until three miscarriages have occurred, and since these tests are usually very limited anyway, this will need to be explained tactfully to avoid raised hopes or future resentments. Some parents will not have begun to think of their developing fetus as a real baby and therefore disposal will be as unimportant to them as, say, the disposal of a superfluous appendix following surgery. Some parents may be repelled and not want to have anything to do with their fetus or with the subsequent disposal, but some parents may want to see their fetus and should be offered the opportunity to do so. For parents who perceive their miscarriage as that of a tiny but real baby, some form of burial or cremation may be essential to answer their needs. Many will not know the legal position concerning a miscarried fetus and therefore their doctor can help by advising them that private burial in the garden or cremation at home is perfectly legal and that such a ceremony, with the erection of a cross or marker of some kind and accompanied by flowers or some other outward gesture, may well be a very helpful course of action to take because it will enable them to acknowledge the reality of what has happened – an essential step for them to take in order to begin to come to terms with their loss.

During his or her visit, it is helpful if the doctor can explain the likely physical and emotional consequences of miscarriage and offer a follow-up appointment. The parents are unlikely to be able to absorb all that is being said when they are so distressed and therefore such information can be repeated when the appointment takes place, by which time it will also be clearer as to whether a D and C is likely to be needed.

Hospital staff

Pain relief

The subject of pain relief is an important one. The labour which precedes miscarriage is an appalling situation because the mother's instinct is to try to keep in the baby which her body is making her force out, despite the knowledge that survival outside will almost certainly be impossible. Because labour is taking place before the mother has had any opportunity to learn about its nature and management (via antenatal or mothercraft classes) she may still be totally ignorant about what happens. Instead of co-operating with the labour, many women may find themselves fighting it, with an intense anger against their own bodies for apparently betraying both them and their baby, especially as it can be so hard to accept that something is wrong with the pregnancy and that the baby needs to be expelled before it is old enough to survive.

Because of the particular circumstances miscarriage, whether early or late, can involve a very painful labour without the consolation of knowing that there will be a baby to hold and love at the end of it all. Midwives (or nurses) and doctors need to listen and respond if a woman who is miscarrying reports that she is experiencing severe pain. They should ensure that suitable pain relief is offered, with a full explanation of the choices and implications involved. It is vital that staff resist any temptation to minimize what is happening or to trivialize the pain. This won't ease or remove such pain, it will simply make the woman feel guilty for feeling it and 'making a fuss' and angry at being unheard. Effective forms of pain relief do exist, the onus is upon staff to let mothers know that the offer is available and to make that offer at the appropriate time. Having stressed the importance of avoiding drugs during pregnancy, pain relief used during labour will not make the baby's situation any worse and may well assist the mother during a very stressful time.

Dilation and curettage operation

To the medical staff, both evacuation of retained products of conception (ERPC) and dilation and curettage (D and C) operations (see p. 27) are straightforward surgical procedures, but to the women concerned they may have major emotional implications. Being told that the pregnancy is no longer viable can be a profound shock, especially where there has been little or nothing in the way of forewarning, and staff will need to be sensitive to the differing responses of women who suddenly find themselves in such an unenviable situation. Some may want an ERPC as quickly as possible because they are so distressed at the realization that they are carrying a dead baby inside them. Others may prefer to wait long enough to adjust to what has happened and make suitable arrangements for those at home before proceeding with the operation. Some find the ERPC or D and C a helpful operation, clearing the way for a successful next pregnancy. To others, such an operation may seem intrusive in every sense, an extra stress at an already stressful time. Fear of an anaesthetic can be very real and women faced with an operation will need reassurance and support. At least the operation may help women to see themselves as a patient for a while, in need of rest and recuperation, instead of expecting too much of themselves, too soon, and it can be one clear-cut way of helping them to recognize that miscarriage has taken place and the pregnancy has ended. This is a very brutal realization, but if nothing else it can enable justified grieving to begin, a necessary first step for it ever to be resolved.

Antenatal staff

Antenatal staff become involved when a problem is diagnosed during a routine check-up. Obviously this is a time of great anxiety for any mother who arrives thinking that all is well and suddenly realizes that something may be wrong. Again, staff can do much to help by giving information and explanation and by comforting and offering any reassurance which can be given.

The most usual step when a possible problem is detected is to arrange for an ultrasound scan, but it is difficult to generalize because the situation varies so much from hospital to hospital and clinic to clinic and much will depend on the particular circumstances at the time and the facilities available. Some antenatal clinics have access to portable scan machines, others might have to issue the mother with an appointments card. Even if a scan can be arranged immediately, using hospital facilities, this often means having to wait beforehand and afterwards in a room full of other pregnant women, which can be very upsetting if the scan shows that the pregnancy has ceased to be viable.

Handled well, the scan can help by clarifying the situation, but handled wrongly, it can simply add to the mother's distress. When those who operate the scans are not permitted to give information to the mothers concerned, this places both them and the mothers in an invidious position.

Thankfully some hospitals are now adopting a more understanding approach by allowing the mother's partner, relative or friend to be present during the scan, and by allowing scan operators to give enough information for the mother to know whether or not the pregnancy is viable. Most mothers are well aware in any case that if they are not shown the baby on the screen and no one points out a heartbeat, then something is evidently wrong. Any support which antenatal staff can offer at such a distressing time will be deeply valued. The mother-to-be who arrived for a routine antenatal check-up will feel bewildered and disorientated if she suddenly finds that she has to have a scan or that she is to become a hospital patient. So, if she needs to be admitted immediately, then it helps if someone from the antenatal clinic can accompany her, not simply to hand over her notes but to give her support as well. Obviously, again, this will depend on staffing levels and when antenatal clinics are very understaffed they may have to rely on porters, but when they can be present, this is of great help.

After the miscarriage

The family doctor

Often it is afterwards that the family doctor can be of most help but it is also the time when he or she may inadvertently do the most harm. Considerate treatment at this time can do much to reduce the trauma and help the woman who has miscarried to recover and to cope. I know from talking with women who have miscarried that the doctors they value most are those who show that they care, especially if they make contact of their own accord by telephoning, visiting or at least offering a follow-up appointment. Some useful Don'ts and Dos to bear in mind are:

Don't compound the woman's own sense of guilt and self-blame by thoughtless remarks such as: 'What a naughty girl! What have you been up to, then?' Trying to trivialize the miscarriage in such a patronizing way is both inappropriate and unfair and will not help the woman concerned at all.

Don't deny the miscarriage by suggesting that the sick note should contain vague information such as 'stomach trouble'. Acknowledge the miscarriage to your patient – it is very real to her – and explain to her that her sick note will be seen by her employer and then let her make the appropriate decision. Most women will want to say what has happened, some may prefer to keep the miscarriage private, but either way the decision should be theirs and not be one which is imposed on them.

Don't minimize the miscarriage. This does not reduce the pain of grieving in any way, it merely makes the woman concerned feel guilty for experiencing such intense emotions over an event which is obviously regarded by others as trivial. Trying to minimize what has happened will impede rather than assist recovery.

Do acknowledge the miscarriage and give the woman concerned full permission to grieve. She may well be trying to deny her grief to herself in an effort to 'get back to normal' as quickly as possible and to conform to the image which others are imposing on her every time they tell her she is 'doing so well'. Being given permission by you to grieve for her loss will allow her to recognize and accept her true feelings and therefore enable her to begin working through them and resolving them.

Do be aware that a woman who has miscarried may afterwards suffer severe depression which she may not even recognize, let alone know how to resolve. It may well be up to you to recognize the signs on her behalf and to encourage her to undertake treatment which she may not even feel is necessary.

Do forewarn both partners of likely grief reactions as this will help them to recognize these reactions and assist them in dealing with the extremes of mood and emotions which may follow a miscarriage. It is very distressing and disorientating to find oneself at the mercy of unexpected and violent feelings and very reassuring to discover that such feelings are perfectly normal and that they will ease in time and pass.

Do be willing to refer patients who have miscarried to professional counselling, if this seems appropriate. It won't always be needed, but it should be offered. If you can keep near at hand details of any support groups in the area, with current telephone numbers of contacts, this could well be one very helpful way of providing your patient with information and support.

Hospital staff

Answering the emotional needs of women who have miscarried will place much greater demands on staff than merely answering their physical needs. These physical needs can be as basic as ensuring the provision of sanitary towels and giving information concerning the location of the nearest toilet and washing facilities. Answering the emotional needs can be much more complex. Immediately after the miscarriage, it is important for staff to allow the woman concerned to retain the power of decisions because this can give her a sense of self-worth and control at a time when both her body and the situation around her seem to be totally out of control. Instead of making decisions on her behalf, ask her (and her partner if he is present) whether they would like to see their baby and resist taking action such as disposal until they have had a chance to become calm and rational enough to make an informed decision on their own behalf. Where staff can help is by, for example, taking a photo of the baby if this is appropriate (usually beyond the 18th week of pregnancy), retaining the photo and informing the parents later that it is available and will remain so, should they wish to see it at a later date.

It is easy to assume that someone else is giving the kind of information that is needed at such a time. If possible, staff should establish a policy whereby they will know for certain that someone will:

1) Inform the parents of the options open to them concerning arrangements for the embryo/fetus/baby who has miscarried
2) Explain what is available in the way of tests on the placental tissue and on the fetus
3) Explain what is available in the way of follow-up treatment for the mother
4) Forewarn the parents of likely grief reactions
5) Give information concerning the Miscarriage Association and any local support group.

It is a very difficult situation, because being in hospital can make a mother who has just miscarried feel out of place but being discharged too soon can leave her feeling abandoned and scared, especially if she then experiences the sort of problems which can follow a full-term birth such as after-pains and contractions, heavy bleeding and engorged breasts. Some hospitals arrange follow-up care, others do not and there seems to be little consistency, although much will depend on the stage of pregnancy reached at the time of the miscarriage and whether the woman was under the antenatal care of her family doctor or the hospital clinic. Even when the mother does receive a follow-up appointment, this can be a mixed blessing. Ideally it should be an opportunity for asking questions and expressing feelings. More often it can become an added cause of distress if the woman concerned encounters a doctor (whether at junior or at consultant level) who has not taken the time to read her notes beforehand and who displays a lack of interest or concern. It is all too easy for doctors who are satisfied with the physical recovery of their patient to underestimate the emotional impact of miscarriage and to fail to recognize the very strong need for an explanation which is felt by most mothers. Whilst accepting that often it is not possible to say why the miscarriage happened, mothers need to know that everything possible has been done to discover the cause. Obviously, if all miscarriages were investigated routinely, then this would completely overstretch the medical staff available and divert help from those who need it most. On the other hand mothers are unlikely to forgive the doctor who obliges them to undergo three miscarriages before initiating investigation and treatment if such investigation and treatment then reveal that the miscarriages were preventable. One woman who wrote to me said:

> I wish they would take time to give more advice and give you time to ask questions. It would be nice if they could give a number of a doctor or midwife you could ring if you have any questions, as I know there are lots I would like to ask but can't.

If the miscarriage is an early one, the hospital is most likely to give the woman a letter to take to her doctor, or to contact the doctor on her behalf. As the family doctor is in a better position than a hospital to know the woman and her home circumstances, a subsequent visit to her doctor is likely to benefit her more than one to the hospital, although again some doctors are unwilling or unable to give their patient the time and attention needed.

Sometimes the cause of the miscarriage can be diagnosed and successfully treated in a straightforward way, but often the picture is unclear and treatments unproven. As mentioned in Chapter 1, surgery can sometimes be successful in correcting an abnormally shaped womb, but the other possible treatments discussed in

Chapter 1 are more contentious. There are mixed views, for example, about the use of hormone supplementation, the role played by immunotherapy treatment and the effectiveness of the cervical stitch, but on the other hand there are women who will testify to the validity of all three and it helps if doctors can be willing to keep an open mind where possible treatments are concerned. If nothing else, offering tangible treatments enables women who have miscarried to know that someone cares enough to do something and may well give them the reassurance and confidence needed to carry the next pregnancy to successful completion.

Hopefully, if more accurate figures can be obtained regarding the extent and frequency of miscarriage and more research financed into the possible causes and possible means of prevention, then the outlook for everyone experiencing miscarriage will improve.

Health visitors, community midwives and antenatal staff

Once miscarriage has taken place, the woman concerned no longer 'qualifies' for antenatal care and so an important pattern in her life abruptly ends. Visits from her health visitor or community midwife, however, can provide her with a much-needed opportunity to talk and to ask questions such as how long the bleeding can be expected to last (it should stop by two or three weeks after the miscarriage). Such support, therefore, should be offered if at all possible.

I began this chapter with a profound awareness of the un-answered needs of parents bereaved by miscarriage. I am able to end it on a note of definite optimism for the future. The fact that a motion concerning the management of miscarriages and stillbirths was debated in the House of Commons in February 1991 is an indication that the needs of mothers who miscarry are beginning to be recognized and given some long-needed attention. In addition, a number of hospitals and crematoriums are beginning to recognize that parents who experience pregnancy loss often feel a strong need to say goodbye to their miscarried babies in an appropriate way and are beginning to take steps to answer that need. Recently I attended the inaugural meeting of the Worthing Crematorium and Cemeteries Liaison Group. I had been invited on behalf of the Miscarriage Association and I went not knowing what to expect. As I drove into the crematorium, it reminded me of the crematorium in Darlington where, 12 years ago, we watched Elizabeth's tiny coffin being carried into the chapel. Immediately I was back there again and shocked to discover the depth of my distress. I stopped the car for a few minutes and sat there thinking: 'Dear God, does this pain never end?' Worthing crematorium is in a large area which has been laid out as a wildlife sanctuary. As I sat watching pheasants cropping contentedly in one of the fields, a sense of peace replaced the pain and I was able to drive on to the meeting, where I was made most welcome. The aim of the meeting was to discover ways of improving customer care and 'care' was the word which dominated. The staff are to be congratulated for initiatives which it is hoped other crematoriums may emulate. Iron entrance gates can look very forbidding. At Worthing Crematorium there are now no gates at all, and at the nearby cemetery the gates are kept permanently open, to enable those at work during the day to visit after working hours if they wish to do so. Everything possible is done to help bereaved families. A wide variety of cassettes means that appropriate music is always available to bereaved families for services, ranging from religious to non-religious, classical to pop and including Chris de Burgh's very moving track, from his *Flying Colours* LP called 'Carry Me (Like a Fire in Your Heart)' which apparently he wrote for friends whose baby had died and which many find comforting following miscarriage, stillbirth, neonatal death or cot death.

A video is available for loan, showing the layout of the large and small chapels as well as the surrounding grounds, so that families can watch it in the privacy of their own homes, familiarize themselves and decide whether cremation is the right option for them.

A special area is set aside for children and babies and, although under no obligation to do so, all the staff are willing to arrange, free of charge, for babies lost before birth to be given a cremation service. The staff also offer facilities to memorialize at the crematorium or cemetery and offer all families the opportunity to make an entry in The Book of Remembrance. All these facilities mean that the staff are giving to babies lost before birth the most important gift of all – acknowledgement. The staff are honest. They know that these babies have no legal recognition and they know that no ashes will remain, but they are sensitive to the deep need which many bereaved parents feel for some acceptable way of saying goodbye to their babies who die before or at birth and in this they have the full co-operation of Worthing hospital.

Some hospitals, such as The Royal Devon and Exeter Hospital in Exeter, now offer subsequent support to parents bereaved by miscarriage. Two months ago I attended the first meeting of a bereavement support group set up by midwives and nurses at Crawley hospital for those experiencing pregnancy loss. They, too, had recognized that, following such a loss, parents need to talk and to know that someone is listening. They have established the group of their own accord and are running it in their own spare time, as a way of showing that they care. Where hospital staff like those at Crawley and crematorium staff like those at Worthing, can set such an encouraging example, hopefully others can and will follow. We may feel that as bereaved parents we are powerless, but the more that we can make our needs known in our own immediate areas, the more chance there is that those needs will be recognized and met.

8

Another Baby?

Whether to try again

Many factors need to be taken into account when deciding whether to try and conceive again, not least the implications for you and your family. If you already have children, they will be aware of some of the effects of your previous miscarriage or miscarriages even if they do not fully understand what you have experienced. Any threat to your health is also a threat to their security, and whilst the prospects for a future successful pregnancy are excellent, these must be weighed against the risk of another miscarriage, more hospitalization, more grieving. Your husband or partner will also be affected by your decision. Having watched you suffer before, he may be very reluctant to risk letting you suffer again and may even, like your children, dread the thought of more disruption. Resting at home or in hospital to try and improve the chances of a successful pregnancy may, even though it is unproven, help any future baby but inevitably it will disrupt family life. So will trying to improve any future baby's chances by altering your dietary intake and lifestyle. Sometimes, without realizing it, the urge to conceive and maintain a pregnancy can come to dominate our whole lives to the detriment both of ourselves and those around us. On the other hand, their needs have to be weighed against our own. If another baby is the only way to answer those needs, then you must be true to your instinct and hopefully, by explaining this to your family, you will be able to enlist their encouragement and support.

Sometimes the strain of miscarriage can contribute to the failure of a relationship, an added grief for both concerned. Some may find themselves without a partner but still with a very deep need for another baby. This can be a very distressing time, but at least it holds out the possibility of happiness in the future, if the couple become reconciled later or if they find a new partner and are able to try again to have a baby. Sadly, for some, a future successful pregnancy may never be possible, if, for example, they have had repeated miscarriages and have been told that their particular problem means that they will never carry a baby to term. Those who have suffered the loss of both of their Fallopian tubes through ectopic pregnancies may still have a chance through *in vitro* fertilization, but after all that they have endured it would take great courage to continue and, of course, *in vitro* fertilization is very expensive and carries no guarantee of a happy outcome. It is an option, though, and a number of couples now exist who can testify to its success.

Adoption remains a possibility for those whose particular history of miscarriage means that they will never be able to bear children of their own and again, adoption can result in great happiness for both the parents and the children concerned, but as there are relatively few babies in the UK available for adoption, not all couples will be accepted, especially if the years spent trying for a baby of their own mean that they are now considered too old by adoption agencies. Life can be very cruel indeed.

Tests and investigations

Having already experienced miscarriage, should you ask to undergo any available medical tests or investigations before risking another pregnancy? As mentioned earlier, most doctors are reluctant to refer couples until three consecutive miscarriages have occurred because they regard miscarriage, with some statistical justification, as a 'self-righting event'. However, anyone who has experienced a 'mid-trimester' (from 14 to 28 weeks) miscarriage should ask to be checked for cervical incompetence, so that, if necessary, a purse-string stitch can be inserted during the next pregnancy (see pp. 104 and 105 for further details).

Even when doctors do make a referral for tests the investigations which can be done at the moment are very limited. Chromosome analysis and genetic counselling, HLA antigen testing for possible immunological problems (see p. 11), blood grouping and checking for rhesus antibodies, testing for infection, hormone estimates, hysterosalpingogram to check for abnormalities of the shape of the uterus or cervical canal – all are possibilities, but none carries any guarantee of success. During any subsequent pregnancy, very little can be done to forewarn of a possible miscarriage. Blood tests can be offered at 16–18 weeks to screen for spina bifida and anencephaly, with further blood tests and a scan if there is doubt, but only four techniques currently exist which can warn of abnormalities in the developing baby which might lead to miscarriage. These are chorionic villus sampling (CVS), amniocentesis, fetoscopy and cordocentesis. These techniques (discussed on p. 15) themselves carry a small risk of triggering miscarriage, and if an abnormality is found, you then face the agonizing decision of whether to terminate the pregnancy or take on the care and responsibility of a baby who, if he or she survives, will be handicapped. The situation is not helped by the fact that false–positives can and do sometimes occur. Thankfully, they are not common but unfortunately the possibility of such an eventuality merely adds to the dilemma already being faced by the parents concerned. Fetoscopy is only available at a few specialized units and it is likely to be superseded by cordocentesis (in which a fine needle is passed through the uterus to where the umbilical cord is joined to the placenta to enable blood to be sampled) as it means that there is no need to insert the larger fetoscope into the uterus and this reduces the risk of miscarriage.

Treatments

Although it in no way reduces our sense of loss, most of us can accept that if our fetus is abnormal, our bodies are right to miscarry. What is far more difficult to accept is the miscarriage of normal fetuses and therefore the urge to seek any treatment which might prevent this is very strong indeed. Sadly, of the tests which can be done at present, few are able to be followed by effective treatment. The tests may provide some answers, but they do not prevent future miscarriage. Possible exceptions to this somewhat depressing realization are:

1) *Immunotherapy* (see p. 12 for further details).
2) *Anti-D-gammaglobulin* injections for women who are rhesus negative and who have had a miscarriage, to prevent the formation of antibodies in the mother's bloodstream which would otherwise try and destroy the next baby's red blood cells.
3) *Antibiotic treatment* for infections which may be linked with miscarriage.
4) *Insertion of a cervical stitch* – the Shirodkar or MacDonald suture. The cervical stitch (suture) can be compared to the drawstring of a purse. Under general or epidural anaesthetic, the stitch is inserted into the neck of the uterus to 'draw it together' and keep it closed during the pregnancy in cases where the cervix is known to be weak and liable to open too soon. Insertion should not be performed after 32 weeks of pregnancy and therefore it is usually

done during the second trimester (weeks 13–24), after the risk of first-trimester miscarriage has passed. Some doctors, however, prefer to insert the stitch early in pregnancy. The stitch is usually removed at 38 weeks of pregnancy, in hospital but without the need for a general anaesthetic. Sometimes removal may trigger contractions or break the waters, leading to labour, but in many cases the pregnancy will continue to the allotted 40 weeks. If labour begins before the stitch has been removed, it is important to notify your doctor immediately, to avoid the risk of serious complications and damage to the uterus. Opinions are divided as to the effectiveness of the stitch as a means of preventing miscarriage. Some medical professionals do not even accept that the condition of cervical incompetence exists, and more evidence is needed (potential researchers please note!). If you would like more details concerning this whole subject, there is a booklet by Ros Kane called *The Cervical Stitch: What It's Like* and there is also support available in the form of the Stitch Network, which offers contact for anyone having or considering this treatment (address at the end of this book).

5) *Hormone treatment.* Here again, opinions are divided. The two female hormones, oestrogen and progesterone, have both been given to women with a history of recurrent miscarriage, but it is now recognized that a synthetic oestrogen used in the USA in the 1950s (stilboestrol) led to a link in the 1970s with vaginal cancer, abnormal reproductive organs and fertility problems in young women whose mothers had used this hormone during pregnancy. Synthetic progestogen preparations are still in use, but again some have been shown to affect the developing labia and clitoris of baby girls, so perhaps they should be used with much more caution, especially since studies suggest that there is no difference in the rate of subsequent miscarriage between using progesterone and using a placebo (the ineffective 'sugar pill'), which implies that any beneficial effect derives from the psychological support of something being done, rather than the something itself.

Another hormone supplement which has been used to try and prevent miscarriage is the pregnancy hormone HCG (human chorionic gonadotrophin), in an attempt to make the corpus luteum produce more natural progesterone, but as so often there are conflicting findings, so more research and evaluation are needed.

6) *Surgery* for uterine abnormalities and fibroids (myomas). If miscarriage is being caused by a uterine abnormality and this is discovered by means of a hysterosalpingogram (see p. 103), then

surgery can usually correct the problem. If fibroids (see p. 6) are thought to be distorting the cavity of the uterus and affecting the ability of the uterus to maintain the pregnancy, then an operation known as a myomectomy can be performed to remove them.

7) *Bed-rest, psychotherapy and good support.* Bed-rest has long been the most common treatment for the prevention of miscarriage, with very little scientific evidence to support it. If the body is trying to miscarry a fetus which is abnormal or dead, then bed-rest will not prevent this necessary process. If, on the other hand, the bleeding is being caused by the placenta detaching itself from the uterine lining, then bed-rest may give the best chance of successful reattachment. Recommending bed-rest at least enables the doctor to feel that he is giving a response and enables the mother to feel that she is doing something positive to save the pregnancy. It has the distinct advantage of being harmless and if the woman feels that she will benefit from it, then she may well do so. Psychotherapy is more common in the USA than in the UK, but results suggest that supporting women in this way can be beneficial. Such treatment begs the whole question of whether a woman's mental and emotional health prior to conception is relevant during pregnancy and as yet studies which can be accurately evaluated are still lacking, but this is an area which may prove useful in the future. The same holds true for simple, straightforward medical support involving frequent personal contact and weekly medical examinations. A study in Norway using this method produced a very high success rate, and although it was not a randomized controlled trial it does perhaps indicate that such treatment does no harm and may well do some good.

When to try again

Most couples who experience miscarriage will want to try for another baby and thankfully most will be able to do so; the difficult decision comes in knowing when the time is right. Much will depend on the nature of the previous miscarriage and at what stage of pregnancy it took place. Many women may find themselves torn between the need to recover fully from the miscarriage and the desire to have another baby as soon as possible. The situation may also arise where one partner wants another baby straightaway but the other wants time to grieve and adjust to what has happened, and this can cause conflict (see also p. 65). As always, good communication will help and explaining your feelings will minimize the risk of misunderstandings or resentments. Even after consulting others and listening to what doctors, relatives and friends have to say, ultimately the decision is one which only you as a couple can make and it should be made with as much tolerance and understanding on both sides as possible.

If you do both wish to go ahead and try for another baby, it is worth remembering that a woman's body can take up to two years to recover fully from the effects of pregnancy and childbirth and that this will apply to late miscarriages just as it does to full-term pregnancies. Few couples would wish to delay for two years, but equally it would be sensible to give consideration to preconceptual care and to endeavour to be as healthy as possible before embarking on another pregnancy. The charity organization Foresight is able to give valuable advice and help in this respect. Having experienced miscarriage once or more, it obviously makes sense to give any subsequent pregnancy the maximum chance of success. This will include checking with your doctor to ensure that you are immune to rubella and it will also include trying to abstain from cigarettes, drugs and alcohol and ensuring a healthy, balanced diet with supplements (if necessary and appropriate) of vitamins and folic acid and of calcium, iron, and other minerals.

Medical advice on how long to wait can range from 'try immediately' to 'wait at least a year' and no one seems to know for certain whether there is a suitable time to wait before trying to conceive again, but research has been done which shows that becoming pregnant again very soon after having a baby increases the risk of the next baby being of low birthweight and that rapid successive pregnancies increase the risk of cot death.

Most doctors recommend that if you have suffered an early miscarriage, you should wait at least three months before trying to conceive again and that if you have suffered a late miscarriage, then you should wait longer. Often women who do wait obediently and then try again expect to conceive straightaway and are deeply disappointed if they encounter delay, but this may simply mean that their bodies are still making hormonal adjustments following the miscarriage or are needing more time to recover. Pregnancy involves great changes in a woman's system – not just her hormone levels but also her biochemistry, circulation and immunology, and it also tends to deplete her of essential nutrients which her body will need to replenish afterwards.

Not conceiving straightaway can reinforce feelings of failure, especially since, as mentioned earlier, the menstrual blood acts as a physical reminder of the miscarriage and all its associations. If you do experience delay (and this is very common), you may well find yourself having to cope with renewed depression every time your period arrives and feel that you are in a kind of limbo, metaphorically holding your breath each month and dreading the sight of any blood every time you go to the toilet. It is a classic no-win situation, because if and when you do become pregnant, you will probably spend the next nine months dreading exactly the same scenario!

As well as needing time to recover physically, you are likely to need time to recover emotionally, and it is important to allow yourself to grieve for the baby you have lost, no matter how early in the pregnancy, before embarking on a new pregnancy. This is because if you become pregnant while you are still grieving you may well find yourself torn between your feelings for the baby who has died and your feelings for the baby who is growing inside you. The natural response is to opt for your growing baby, but this can lead you to suppress your grieving and suppressed, unresolved grieving has a habit of re-emerging later.

One other important point should be considered before deliberately trying to have another baby and that is the possible implications for you and your partner when making love. For most couples, lovemaking is an end in itself and not merely a means to an end. As stressed in Chapter 5 (see p. 65), there is a danger when desperately wanting to conceive that lovemaking will be reduced to simply a mechanical means to an end, with the woman only wanting to make love at the 'right' time of month, around the time of ovulation, and the man as a consequence feeling used instead of feeling loved. It helps if you can continue to regard your lovemaking as a pleasure in its own right, with any subsequent pregnancy coming as an added bonus. You may also need to be prepared for feelings of intense protectiveness towards the developing baby once you do conceive, which may make you reluctant to make love during pregnancy in case it poses a potential threat. With the possible avoidance of a few specific occasions (see p. 9), there is no evidence to suggest that lovemaking places the baby at risk in any way. Lovemaking towards the very end of pregnancy may stimulate the cervix and thereby release hormones which initiate labour, but that is an entirely different matter, though worth remembering if your baby is overdue!

Having a miscarriage can be a profound blow to our whole image of ourselves and our understanding of our femininity. Many of us decide to have a baby because it seems the obvious and natural course of action when the time is appropriate, which is usually within the emotional and financial security of marriage or a stable, loving relationship. We probably do not think through all the implications and it is unlikely that we anticipate any real problems. With hindsight, such confidence and such innocent assumptions that all will be well can seem cruelly naive. Experiencing a miscarriage presents us with some very stark realities concerning our mortality, our vulnerability, our limitations. At the same time as we are forced to recognize that we cannot take future motherhood for granted, we often also suddenly realize just how important motherhood is to us: with miscarriage, we lose both our baby and our motherhood. Many of us may find ourselves having to cope with a very deep need to 'prove' ourselves both to ourselves and to others, to show that we are capable of motherhood, and such a realization can come as a shock and a complete revelation.

Common anxieties and reactions

Not everyone experiences the problem of anxiety during their subsequent pregnancy, so please don't feel guilty if you're enjoying it, or start worrying because you're not worrying! It is very encouraging to know that some women *are* able to enjoy their pregnancies and have a trouble-free time. The reason for mentioning likely anxieties and reactions is to forewarn and forearm those who may find themselves having to cope with such eventualities while they are pregnant. During the early weeks, before you are seen in the antenatal clinic, if you are feeling anxious it is worth contacting your community midwife (if one is available in your area) or your local health visitor, for advice and reassurance.

One of the most common anxieties concerns bleeding in early pregnancy. I have already mentioned that women who have experienced miscarriage are likely to spend part or all of their next pregnancy looking for signs of bleeding every time they use the toilet. This is a very natural and understandable reaction, but in the unlikely event of finding some blood on the toilet tissue, what should you do? (It is worth noting that there is very little association between bleeding in pregnancy and any increased risk of abnormality. If the bleeding passes, all should be well.) For peace of mind, however, it makes sense to contact your doctor, even if realistically there is little that he can offer you in the way of treatment. If nothing else, you are alerting him to the possibility of another miscarriage and he in turn may be able to reassure you about the number of pregnancies which do show some bleeding in the early stages and yet go on to be totally successful. At such a time, it is best to follow your instinct. If you feel that you should rest, then do so. If you feel that you should carry on as normal, then likewise you should do so. It is very difficult to stay calm at such a time, but the more that you can practise relaxation during your pregnancy, the more that both you and your baby will benefit. There is evidence to show that the blood flow to the womb increases during times of relaxation, so it is worth learning about relaxation techniques and buying a tape to which you can listen at home.

Good support from your doctor and a feeling of trust in him or her is essential, so if you truly feel that your doctor is unsympathetic and that you cannot relate to each other in any way, then you may wish to consider changing to another, but you should bear in mind that there will be a resultant loss of continuity of care and knowledge of your previous medical history. Good support from your partner, family and friends is also essential, but they may not always be able to answer your needs. The people who are most likely to understand and identify with what you are feeling during your subsequent pregnancy are members of your nearest Miscarriage Association group, because they will have been there, too. It can be very reassuring to find that unexpected reactions which you had thought were unique to yourself can in fact be very common and that you are perfectly normal!

Miscarriage can raise many anxieties because it undermines self-confidence. A traumatic miscarriage may leave you fearing the pain of a subsequent labour more than you otherwise might have done, because you know from experience that things can go wrong. During your next pregnancy you may also find yourself worrying more than others would about the risk of handicap, stillbirth or cot death. Since your plans have already gone wrong before, you are bound to be aware that they could go wrong again, but try to remember that this does not mean that they will do so. The statistics are all in your favour.

It is only natural to feel worried or depressed at times during a subsequent pregnancy, but if there are times when you feel that you will never succeed in having a baby and never know the fulfilment of motherhood, then try quoting the relevant statistics to yourself because they really are reassuring. There is always a 15–20 per cent risk of miscarriage with any pregnancy, so those who have never had a miscarriage have an 80–85 per cent chance of a normal pregnancy. You have been one of the unlucky ones, but try to remember that after one miscarriage you still have a 75 per cent chance of having a normal pregnancy and that is very high. Even if you are very unlucky and have had two, three or even four miscarriages, you still have a 68 per cent chance of a normal pregnancy next time and that's very encouraging. Obviously much will depend on what has caused the single or recurrent miscarriage. If the cause was chromosomal abnormality, you are less likely to miscarry the second time because this tends to happen by chance, whereas if the reason is hormonal, structural or an infection, then it is more likely to go on causing problems until it is treated. The one exception where chromosome abnormality is concerned is where there is a chromosomal abnormality which for some reason keeps recurring in the fetus (which is very rare) or where the parents have chromosomal abnormalities in their own cells which they then pass on to their fetus. This genetic problem, known as balanced translocation, only occurs in about 5 per cent of couples and tests are available to confirm whether or not it is the case. However unlikely it may seem at the time, miscarriage *is*, as the doctors so clinically phrase it, usually a 'self-righting condition'.

One common reaction during a subsequent pregnancy is to refuse to make any preparations or to allow ourselves to enjoy the pregnancy for fear of 'tempting fate'. Refusing to acknowledge the coming baby is one way of trying to protect ourselves from the risk of pain and disappointment, though it can cause problems later (see p. 112). It is very sad that having a miscarriage can destroy what should be the excitement and fulfilment of pregnancy. Few can ever relax or take a subsequent pregnancy for granted. In losing our baby we lose also a sense of innocence. When chatting to others at antenatal clinics or classes we can feel embarrassed because we are the bad news which no one wants to hear and we may well feel that we have to protect them and not destroy their confidence and innocence as well. I can remember going to the clinic when I was expecting Christopher and sitting next to a very young and happy first time mother-to-be. 'How many children have you had?' she asked eagerly and I couldn't do it to her so I just answered: 'Two, both girls', in my mind feeling that I was betraying our first baby and our twin daughter Elizabeth by not acknowledging them and mentally apologizing and explaining to them why I could not do so.

Another common reaction is to restrict ourselves as much as possible in the hope that this will improve the chances of a successful pregnancy. Some women almost punish themselves, giving up what they enjoy most as an unspoken offering to an unknown fate, an appeasement to protect their unborn child. We blame ourselves for the previous miscarriage or miscarriages and play the 'if only' game – 'if only I hadn't gone on working'; 'if only I hadn't gone on holiday'. It's an understandable reaction, but it isn't necessary. Unless specifically advised not to do so, you should carry on as normal.

Success!

After all the grief of the previous miscarriage and all the waiting and stress of the next pregnancy, when the new baby does arrive it is as well to be prepared for a strange feeling of anticlimax. If you have been consciously or unconsciously distancing yourself from your baby during pregnancy as a protection against the pain of another possible miscarriage, then it can take some time to relax and adjust to your baby and begin to believe in him or her as a reality. Many mothers, especially if they have had to cope with recurrent miscarriage, feel that the baby won't stay, that he or she is merely on loan and will be snatched away if they dare to give too much love. Allow yourself time to recognize that your baby *is* real and with you to stay and accept that it may take a while before you are able to enjoy your baby and risk acknowledging and showing your love.

Some women suffer postnatal depression, and then compound their problem by feeling guilty at not being able to enjoy the baby they have wanted for so long. If this happens, be patient with yourself, talk to your doctor or midwife, and allow your hormone levels time to return to normal. Try to remember that these feelings will pass and that once they do, the love will flow and the deep and lasting happiness of motherhood will be able to begin.

Not everyone experiences a sense of anticlimax or a form of postnatal depression. With luck you will be able to enjoy your baby from the moment of birth onwards. Miscarriage changes us, we can never be the same as we were before it happened, but once you have your baby you are less likely to be trapped by your previous history of miscarriage and it is less likely to dominate your life or overwhelm you, because you will find that sooner or later you will be able to place it in context. Very few of us ever forget, but in time it becomes possible to acknowledge the place that miscarriage has in our lives, to learn to live with that acknowledgement and then to allow ourselves to move on and be open to whatever the future holds.

Useful Addresses

United Kingdom

AIMS (Association for Improvements in Maternity Services)
40 Kingswood Avenue
London NW6
Tel: 081 960 5585

ASBAH (Association for Spina Bifida and Hydrocephalus)
ASBAH House
42 Park Road
Peterborough, PE1 2UQ
Tel: 0733 555988

Birthright
27 Sussex Place
London NW1 4SP
Tel: 071 723 9296/262 5337

The British Association of Counselling
1 Regent Place
Rugby CV21 2PJ
Tel: 0788 578328

British Association of Psychotherapists
47 Mapesbury Road
London NW2 4HJ
Tel: 081 452 9823

British Diabetic Association
10 Queen Anne Street
London W1M 0BD
Tel: 071 323 1531

The Compassionate Friends
6 Denmark Street
Clifton
Bristol BS1 5DQ
Tel: 0272 292778

Cruse
Cruse House
126 Sheen Road
Richmond
Surrey TW9 1UR

Endometriosis Association
65 Holmdene Avenue
London SE24 9LD
Tel: 071 737 4764

Foresight (The Association for the Promotion of Preconceptual Care)
The Old Vicarage
Church Lane
Witley
Godalming
Surrey GU8 5PN
Tel: 0428 794500

Issue (Formerly the National Association for the Childless)
318 Summer Lane
Birmingham B19 3RL
Tel: 021 359 4887

Listeria Society
Hewshott Farm
Hewshott Lane
Liphook
Hampshire GU30 7SU
Tel: 0428 723100

The Maternity Alliance
15 Britannia Street
London WC1X 9JP
Tel: 071 837 1265

The Miscarriage Association
c/o Clayton Hospital
Northgate
Wakefield
West Yorkshire WF1 3JS
Tel: 0924 200799 (24 hr answerphone)

National Childbirth Trust
Alexandra House
Oldham Terrace
London W3 6NH
Tel: 081 992 8637

Perinatal Bereavement Unit
The Adult Department
Tavistock Clinic
Belsize Park
London NW3 5BA
Tel: 071 435 7111

Relate (Formerly Marriage Guidance)
Listed locally in telephone directories
Head Office:
Herbert Gray College
Little Church Street
Rugby CV21 3AP
Tel: 0788 573241

SANDS (Stillbirth and Neonatal Death Society)
28 Portland Place
London W1N 3DE
Tel: 071 436 5881

SATFA (Support After Termination For Abnormality)
29–30 Soho Square
London W1V 6JB
Tel: 071 439 6124

Sickle Cell Society
54 Station Road
Harlesden
London NW10 4UA
Tel: 081 961 4006

The Stitch Network
Fairfield
Wolverton Road
Norton Lindsey
Warwickshire CV35 8NA
Tel: 092 684 3223

USEFUL ADDRESSES

TAMBA (Twins And Multiple Births Association)
c/o Mrs Sheila Payne
59 Sunnyside
Worksop
North Nottinghamshire
Tel: 0786 72080

Toxoplasmosis Trust
61–71 Collier Street
London N1 9BE
Tel: 071 713 0663

V.D.U. Workers' Rights Campaign
c/o City Centre
32–35 Featherstone Street
London EC1Y 8QX

WHRICC (Women's Health and Reproductive Rights Information
  Centre)
52–54 Featherstone Street
London EC1Y 8RT
Tel: 071 251 6580

United States of America

Resolve Through Sharing
Lutheran Hospital – La Crosse
1910 South Avenue
La Crosse
Wisconsin 54601
Tel: (608) 785 0530

Australia

The Miscarriage Support Group of Australia
PO Box 633
Willoughby
NSW 2068

Canada

Born to Love
21 Potsdam Road
Unit 61
Downsview
Ontario M3N 1N3
Tel: (416) 663 7143

New Zealand

SANDS
c/o Mr and Mrs C. G. Ferguson
30 Church Street
Palmerston North

Further reading

This list of books for further reading is by no means comprehensive, but it includes those books which I or others known to me have found useful.

Beech, Beverley Lawrence. *Who's Having Your Baby?* Bedford Square Press/NCVO, 1991.

Borg, Susan and Lasker, Judith. *When Pregnancy Fails,* Routledge and Kegan Paul, 1983.

Bourne, Gordon. *Pregnancy* (pp. 265–81), Pan, 1984.

Bradford, Nikki. *The Well Woman's Self-Help Directory,* Sidgwick and Jackson, 1990.

Hampshire, Susan. *The Maternal Instinct,* Sphere, 1984.

Hey, Valerie, Catherine Itzin, Lesley Saunders, and Mary Anne Speakman. *Hidden Loss,* The Women's Press, 1989.

Hill, Susan. *Family* (an autobiography), Penguin, 1989.

Huisjes, H. J. *Spontaneous Abortion,* Churchill Livingstone, 1984.

Huws, Ursula. *Visual Display Unit Hazards Handbook: A Worker's Guide to the Effects of New Technology,* London Hazards Trust, 1987.

Jones, Wendy. *Miscarriage: Overcoming the Physical and Emotional Trauma,* Thorsons, 1990.

Kane, Ros. *The Cervical Stitch: What It's Like,* Miscarriage Association, available from the Stitch Network, 1986.

Lachelin, G. C. L. *Miscarriage: The Facts,* Oxford University Press, 1985.

Leroy, Margaret. *Miscarriage,* Optima, 1988.

Morrow, Judy Gordon and DeHamer, Nancy Gordon. *Good Mourning,* Word UK Ltd, 1989.

Moulder, Christine. *Miscarriage,* Pandora, 1990.

Oakley, Ann, Ann McPherson, and Helen Roberts. *Miscarriage,* Penguin, 1990.

Peppers, Larry and Knapp, Ronald. *Motherhood and Mourning, Perinatal Death,* Praeger, 1980.

Phillips, Angela and Rakusen, Jill. *The New Our Bodies Ourselves,* Penguin, 1989.

Pizer, Hank and Palinski, Christine O'Brien. *Coping with a Miscarriage,* Jill Norman, 1980.

Seiden, Othniel. *Coping with Miscarriage,* Tab Books, 1985.

Index

abortion: complete 19;
   incomplete 19, 27; induced 14,
   18, 19, 50; inevitable 19; missed
   19–20; recurrent 20; septic 20;
   spontaneous 18, 19; threatened
   19
accidents 14, 15
adoption 103
age of parents 7, 8
AIDS 11
alcohol 8, 89
alphafetoprotein 16
amniocentesis 15, 104
amniotic fluid 37, 105
anaemia 35
anaesthetic 12, 34, 94, 104–5
anatomical abnormalities 6, 98
anencephaly 16, 103
anger, feelings of 43, 46–9, 54, 62,
   64
antenatal care 17, 89–91, 94–5; see
   also hospital care
antibiotics 10, 34, 104
anti-D gammaglobulin 104

bacterial cause 10
balanced translocation 5, 111
bed-rest 23, 25, 102, 106
Birthright 82, 89, 114
bleeding: afterwards 27, 30, 33,
   34, 97, 99; beforehand 21–2, 24,
   29, 32, 108, 109–10; spotting 19,
   20, 21
blighted ovum 18, 43
blood transfusion 22, 30
breast engorgement 27, 97
breast tenderness 2, 23, 29
brucellosis 10
burial 18, 25, 58, 92

cervical incompetence 6, 14, 103,
   104
cervical stitch 6, 82, 99, 104–5

children 51–2, 68–71, 78, 102
chlamydia 10
choriocarcinoma 32–3
chorionic villus sampling (CVS)
   15, 103
chromosomal abnormalities 4–6,
   111
coil see IUD
colleagues 79–81
community midwife or nurse 89–
   90, 99, 109
conceiving 55, 102, 106–8
confidence, loss of 51–2, 109
contraception 13–14, 34
cordocentesis 15, 104
corpus luteum 105
counselling 82, 96
cremation 25, 99
cytomegalovirus (CMV) 10

D and C (dilation and curettage)
   14, 20, 27, 93–4
denial 42–4, 55, 57, 79, 95, 111–12
depression 34, 42, 45–6, 54–5, 64–
   4, 96, 112
diabetes 11
diagnosis 20–6, 86
diet 13, 89, 102, 107
diethylstilboestrol see stilboestrol
discharge from hospital 43, 97
disorganization, feelings of 45–55
Down's Syndrome 5
dreams about miscarriage 44
drugs, as cause of miscarriage 8,
   89

ectopic pregnancy 13, 28–31, 102–
   3
egg see ovum
embryo 17, 25
emptiness, feelings of 42–3
environmental factors 12
Ergometrine 22

erosion 21
ERPC 27, 93–4

failure, feelings of 51–4, 108
Fallopian tubes 13, 28, 30, 31, 102
falls, as cause of miscarriage 14–15
family doctor 23, 25, 35, 46, 78–9, 85–101
family, effect on 61–71
fear, feelings of 52, 86, 94, 109–10
fertility 9
fertilization 2, 4–5
fetoscopy 15, 104
fetus 11, 17, 25, 57, 92
fever, as cause of miscarriage 10
fibroids (myomas) 6
follow-up care 32–3, 35, 95–101
Foresight 9, 89, 107
friends 66, 69, 72–8
funeral see burial, cremation

GP see family doctor
genetic counselling 5, 103, 111
German measles see rubella
God, feelings about 46–8, 83
grief 41–84, 96, 102, 108
guilt 4, 15, 23, 46, 48–9, 57, 61, 62, 64, 95, 109, 112

habitual miscarriage see recurrent
health-care professionals see hospital care
health visitors 89–90, 99
herpes 11
high blood pressure 11, 32
HIV 11
HLA 12
human chorionic gonadotrophin 7, 26, 105
hydatidiform mole 31–3
hysterosalpingogram 6, 103, 105

illness, as cause of miscarriage 10–11
immunotherapy 11–12, 99, 103
infection, risk of 27, 30, 34
infertility 55
IUD 13, 28–9, 34
in vitro fertilization 31, 103
irradiation 12

labour 24, 27, 40, 53, 91, 93
laparoscopy 30
laparotomy 30
legal definitions 17–18
lifting, as cause of miscarriage 15
listeriosis 10, 115
luteinizing hormone 7

MacDonald suture 104
memorials, mourning rituals 57–9, 92, 100
midwives see hospital care
milk, production of 27–8, 43
miscarriage: at home 23, 24; causes of 3–16; children's reactions to 51, 68–71; definition of 17–18; incidence of 2, 111; in hospital 23, 24, 37–40, 85–9, 93–5, 97–8; research on (and lack of) 2, 5, 105, 106; signs/symptoms of 20–3; treatment of 6–7, 10–12, 22–4 25–8, 52–3, 92, 98–9, 103–6; types of 18–20
Miscarriage Association 3, 18, 82, 115
missed abortion 19–20, 43
molar pregnancy 31–3
morning sickness 2, 23
mycoplasma 10

naming the lost baby 57
NCT 3, 18, 82, 89, 116
nightmares 44
nurses 37–40, 85, 87–91, 93–5, 97–8, 100–1

occupation, as cause of miscarriage 12–13
oestrogen 105
ovary 28, 30
ovulation 34, 108
ovum 4, 5, 17, 28, 31

pain 22, 29, 34, 37, 38, 53, 72, 93, 97
partner 8–9, 52, 61–6, 78, 95, 97, 102, 106–7
pelvic inflammatory disease 10, 28

periods 21, 29, 34–5, 36, 49, 62,
  107–8
pill, the 13, 34
placebo 7, 105
placenta 6, 7, 21, 31, 106
polycystic ovaries 7
polyp 21
preconceptual care 8–9, 13, 89,
  107
pregnancy: feelings during 9, 77,
  108–12; spacing between 51–2,
  107–8; symptoms of 19, 20, 23,
  29
pregnant women, feelings towards
  46, 49, 77–8
privacy, need for 42, 76, 87–8
products of conception 19
progesterone 29
progestogen 7, 13, 105
psychotherapy 83, 106, 114

radioimmunoassay test 29
recovery 56–60
recurrent miscarriage 12, 54–5, 112
relatives 66–9, 72–8
rubella 10

salpingectomy 30
SANDS 18, 116, 118
SATFA 18, 116
salpingo-oopherectomy 30
sanitary towels 30, 33
saying goodbye to your baby 42–4,
  48, 57–9, 92, 99–101
scan see ultrasound scan
'scrape' see D and C
seeing the baby 25, 39, 57–8, 92
sex of the baby 35, 57
sexual intercourse 9, 30, 34, 61–2,
  65, 108
Shirodkar suture 104
shock 42, 86, 93, 109
smoking 8–9, 89

sperm 4, 8, 9, 31
spina bifida 6, 16, 103
spotting see bleeding
stilboestrol 105
stillbirth 17–18, 99, 100
stitch see cervical stitch
stress 8, 15, 109–10
support & lack of 3, 7, 23, 33, 40,
  48, 63, 66–8, 72–101, 106, 110
support groups 3, 81, 96, 101, 110
syphilis 11
Syntocinon 22

termination see abortion, induced
termination after fetal abnormality
  104
tests 25, 103
thyroid problems 11
toxic agents 12
toxoplasmosis 10–11
tranquillizers 42
tubal pregnancy see ectopic
Turner's Syndrome 5
twins 44

ultrasound scan 15, 20, 26, 58,
  94–5
uncertainty, period of 21
ureaplasma 10
uterus 6, 13, 32

VDUs 13, 117
vacuum aspiration 20
vaginal examinations 9, 26
virus infections 10–11

waters breaking 37–8, 105
womb see uterus
work, in pregnancy 12–13
work, return to 79–81

X-rays 12, 26